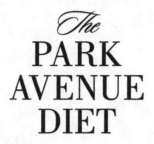

The
PARK
AVENUE
DIET

CHANGE FOR A LIFETIME OF BEAUTY AND HEALTH

The
PARK
AVENUE
DIET

THE COMPLETE 7-POINT PLAN

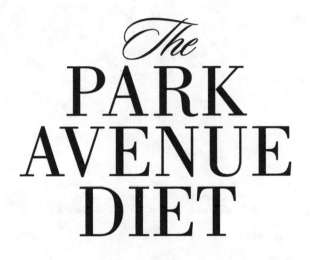

STUART FISCHER, M.D.
FOUNDER OF *THE PARK AVENUE DIET* CENTER

Hatherleigh Press
New York

Hatherleigh Press
5-22 46th Avenue, Suite 200
Long Island City, NY 11101
www.hatherleighpress.com

CIP data available upon request.

ISBN 978-1-57826-263-2
The Park Avenue Diet is available for bulk purchase, special promotions, and premiums.
For information on reselling and special purchase opportunities,
call 1-800-528-2550 and ask for the Special Sales Manager.

Interior design by Maria E. Torres, Neuwirth & Associates, Inc.
Cover design by Christopher Tobias

10 9 8 7 6 5 4 3 2 1
Printed in the United States

ACKNOWLEDGMENTS

The creation of *The Park Avenue Diet,* by its very nature, has been a team effort from the start, led by Richard Rubenstein, whose foresight, support, and creativity have been essential to this project. I deeply appreciate his devotion and wisdom. My superb literary colleagues, Carolyn Fireside, Andrea Au, and Kevin Moran, have been generous with their insights, supervision, and time. What began as professional relationships has blossomed into friendships.

I am also indebted to Kristina Donaj Djelosevic, an assistant of remarkable organizational skills and empathy. Her warmth, patience, and steadfastness have sustained and inspired me for seven years.

Also intrinsic to the success of this project have been the legal counsel of William F. Fitzgerald, a brilliant and caring associate, and the efforts of Bettina Klinger, a marketing expert of rare warmth and dynamism.

I am also truly lucky to have friends such as Seymour Reich, Dr. Edward Arsura, Allan Seif, and Noel Berggren, wonderful relationships that have brightened my life for decades. Thank you one and all.

This book is dedicated to R. Houston Hearn:
photojournalist, humanitarian, and friend.

CONTENTS

PART III
THE PARK AVENUE RECIPES

INTRODUCTION:
CONFESSIONS OF A DIET DOCTOR

*I*n the beginning, looks didn't make a difference. You didn't need to pay attention to your hairstyle, skincare, or clothing choices. You didn't need interpersonal skills either when your enemies were the entire animal kingdom and the sometimes violent forces of nature. When confronted with a snarling animal, you needed a modicum of self-confidence, two strong legs, and lots of energy. Life was simpler.

Eventually, civilization took place, perhaps reaching its all-time peak with the ancient Greeks. They loved sports, theater, sculpture, wine, philosophy, and even healthcare. Moreover, they knew what a lifestyle was, and they had a special name for the concept: *diaitasthai*—"to lead one's life."

Maybe you recognize the first few letters from packages of special frozen food or chemically seasoned dessert dishes. But be assured that you have never thought of the word "diet" the way it was originally conceived.

A lifestyle is one's customary day-by-day pattern of thinking, feeling, decision-making and behaving. Your lifestyle is made visible to the outside world by your image. Your image, in turn, is evident in your appearance and your behavior. These are the twin indicators of who we are, why we act the way we do, and, to a significant extent, how long we are going to live. They also help to determine how much we weigh.

Maybe you thought you knew everything about yourself. Maybe you've come to accept a lifestyle that is not as exciting as one you could really have. Maybe you thought that simply by eating a little less, you'd lose weight—and simply by losing weight, you'd feel more confident, look more attractive, and be more desirable. It doesn't work that way.

May I have the distinct pleasure of showing you how to upgrade your image and, therefore, your lifestyle? You'll need a little extra time every day. You may have to do a little introspection. You'll need to be open to a wide range of new ways to approach old, stale ideas. You'll look much better and feel much happier. In addition, the process will be tremendously enjoyable and fascinating at the same time. And yes, you will lose weight.

But for now, let's turn back the clock a few decades. My approach to upgrading your image was developed several decades ago, although I hardly started out as a role model. Allow me to explain.

I FEEL YOUR GAIN

Here's an autobiographical message to the 66.3 % of Americans now struggling with overweight bodies: I feel your gain.

For too many years, decades ago, I was an expert in obesity as a witness for the prosecution. Patients, colleagues, and friends cannot believe that I was ever overweight. But photographs exist, and since I have definitively corrected the problem I can look back at the "old me" with accrued wisdom.

In fact it's possible I'd still be carrying around those extra 30 to 40 pounds today were it not for an outspoken dose of withering reality from a young medical student named Stuart Fischer who looked at me in the mirror and told me that I needed to change my appearance, image, and interpersonal skills.

That momentous realization would ultimately lead me to devise a weight loss regimen for myself, one which entailed not only shedding pounds but also polishing my personality to match my trim, high-energy body. That was 35 years ago. Since then, I've maintained both my ideal weight and my vastly improved self-image without suffering, starving, living on celery, taking antidepressants, or relapsing. Having ended my weight problem, I want to share with you my remarkably rewarding journey from sloth and self-indulgence to slimness and self-content.

We Baby Boomers who grew up in the fifties were the first generation of children exposed to hypnotically effective television commercials that pushed processed food, refined flour and sugar, cereal additives, and food dyes. How could we resist? Our family had a Saturday night subscription series to the New York Philharmonic; but classical music meant nothing to me at the time, so I concentrated on dinner. Before the concert we would feast at Manhattan restaurants legendary for their gargantuan portions— either Mamma Leone's (where "abbondanza" meant 3 to 4 pounds of food), Luchow's (similar, but Germanic), or a New York steakhouse; the restaurants may be gone but the fat cells remain. Three hours later on our way home, we stopped at Katz's Delicatessen for my "nightcap" corned beef sandwich and a bag of greasy fried potatoes.

Then there was the matter of athletics. I admit in all modesty that my prowess on the 1960s sports field has yet to be equaled by any major medical authority: nobody up to now has ever been as terrible. Although this was the era of President Kennedy's program to improve physical fitness in adolescents, I was unable to perform one chin-up, one push-up or one deep knee-bend. I was able to do a few sit-ups, but only up to a 45-degree angle. To the amazement of my coach (I apologize, Mr. Carney), I ran the quarter-mile in $6^1/_2$ minutes (that's the equivalent of a 26-minute mile, which is slower than walking).

Freshman year at Yale University in 1968 only made my situation worse. I failed a mandatory fitness exam and fainted after a few minutes of an aerobic workout called the Harvard Test (poor choice of a name, by the way) but it didn't matter much. Because athletic credits were not mandatory in the liberal arts program, I spent not one minute in the gym but countless hours in the Morse College dining hall.

This was no run-of-the-mill institutional cafeteria! Students from the Culinary Institute of America did the cooking; and for $1.85 per dinner, fortunate undergrads could enjoy unlimited servings of chicken Cordon Bleu, lobster, filet mignon, and countless other delicacies. Then we would linger over several desserts, downing a few liters of soda, as we engaged in intellectual banter. It was fun. It was fattening. And it was not the only venue in which I could indulge my appetite.

Whenever I traveled from New Haven to New York City for an evening of theater or music, I always dropped by the Sixth Avenue Deli for my all-time favorite snack: a triple-decker combination corned beef/pastrami sandwich, fried potatoes, fried onion rings, cherry cheesecake, and two cream sodas. Try that before a five-hour Wagnerian opera! After the performance, I would buy Taystee Cakes and Oreos from the candy counter at the Port Authority Bus Terminal. Why should I starve myself on the ride back to New Haven?

In 1971, my doctor advised me to go on a diet. His entire recommendation: "learn to like salads." My interpretation: several pounds of vegetables, cheese and meats, topped by an entire jar of Aunt Millie's Blue Cheese Dressing. Despite an Ivy League education, I had no idea why I wasn't losing weight.

Life and my eating habits proceeded in this fashion for another few years. Then one day in 1973 while weighing myself I noticed that my feet had entirely disappeared from view. I looked at myself in the mirror and realized that it was useless to ask my own physician for guidance. Weight loss was not simply about choosing the right food. As a shy "loner" I had totally neglected my personal appearance and become excessively withdrawn. I had to refashion myself internally and externally. I had never cared what people saw when they talked to me, thus isolating myself in an unhealthy and unhappy body. The time had come to reverse the process.

BENNO BLIMPIE

Many years ago I saw a terrific play by the brilliant dramatist Albert Innaurato starring a Yale friend of mine, Peter Evans. It was called *The Transfiguration of Benno Blimpie* and told the story of an unhappy and unloved obese teenager who was constantly tormented and humiliated by his peers. At the end of the play, he was magically changed into a handsome thin man. The actor was wearing a "fat suit," and in the final scene he unzipped it and stepped into the spotlight as his healthy, glamorous self.

I've always felt that inside an overweight man or woman is a thin one trapped by multiple layers of padding. When I first started working with Dr. Robert Atkins and began observing obese people walking down the street, I would look at their round, puffy, pasty faces and would try to imagine what the underlying structures really looked like. But when I observed the residents and professional people on Park Avenue, "all put together" in appearance and behavior, I realized that various components of image—not just weight—work together to create a spectacular whole. And with that realization, the concept of *The Park Avenue Diet* was born.

Of course, I know the subject of weight loss as both a physician and a former "slob"—Dr. Atkins's pithy description of me after glancing at a 1972 photograph. Not only were my eating habits foolish and irresponsible; my clothing, hair, posture and gait were also turn-offs. Not only did my low self-esteem worsen my appearance; my appearance revealed my lack of self-esteem to everyone around. In effect, I was wearing a "fat suit" just like Benno Blimpie.

Reflecting on those years and mistakes, I learned a basic truth. Self-improvement must work in two directions simultaneously: "Inside-out" and "outside-in." Remember this concept. We'll be returning to it often.

THE PARK AVENUE PRINCIPLE

As you probably know from firsthand experience, most people who try to lose weight on typical American fad (food-based) diets inevitably fail. In fact, the cure rate of obesity is the same as the cure rate of lung cancer, 5%, a dismal statistic. All fad diets treat the symptoms but not the cause. This is not unlike a physician's prescribing aspirin for a fever without knowing its source (whether bronchitis, lymphoma, appendicitis, or an allergic reaction). Superficially, the ailing patient feels better although the underlying problem has not been addressed. Do you really think that simply having a different belt size is the path to enlightenment? If so, you've bought into Mistake Number One—*believing that weight loss has magical transformative powers*—and need a thorough re-education in human biochemistry and behavior.

Good looks and longevity, like lasting weight loss, require long-term commitment. More importantly, a pathway to better health and appearance needs to encompass physical, psychological, and behavioral changes that buttress and reinforce each other.

I didn't lose weight or keep it off for the subsequent 35 years merely by eating low-calorie meals for a few months. I had to completely re-invent myself as the slim person inside of me, and that's what you're going to do.

Why do athletes, actors, models, politicians, newscasters, socialites, those fortunate few who comprise the A-list, maintain their svelte appearance in a swirl of constant temptation? Because they have to. Their image, their standing in society, demands discipline, poise, and allure in every aspect of public life, from weight management through social skills to grooming. You must have noticed that the people who have the most money, leisure time, and access to gourmet food, the so-called "idle rich," are virtually never overweight. They know that image dictates diet; the diet does not create an image.

Here's the principle behind my plan: You need to addresses multiple components of image simultaneously. If you focus only on weight loss but wear the same schleppy clothes as always, it's just a matter of time before your taste buds lure you right back to into your fat suit. Similarly, if you weigh a little less but have poor conversational skills, you won't meet the people who could make your life more exciting and will probably revert to your bad habits of spending parties hovering over the buffet table.

NOBODY EVER WON AN INNER BEAUTY CONTEST

If you could create the man or woman of your dreams, what would he or she look like—overweight or thin? Unless you have a fetish for Wagnerian opera singers, being overweight is not an idealized state. Being thin is always preferred. With this single attribute, have we defined your ideal special someone yet? Of course not. Magnetic looks that stop traffic and stimulate hormones are never defined by poundage or any other isolated physical characteristic.

When you imagine what your ideal someone looks like, you'll be captivated by his or her hair, eyes, clothing, physique, smile, conversation, and body language. Every detail registers, whether obviously or subliminally. He or she looks "put together" and usually radiates self-confidence in a unique way—a demure grace, a bravura swagger, a coltish exuberance—as if wearing a neon sign that says "look at me." On the other hand, you don't have to go very far to see someone whose sign reads "I don't care what I look like, so why should you?"

Although we prefer to think that "looks are deceiving" or "you can't judge a book by its cover," your exterior-self is always the first impression made on your neighbors, family, friends, business associates, and even total strangers. Nobody ever won an inner beauty contest. And just as a serious medical illness can often make itself known by visible signs (jaundice, paleness, and rashes), your self-concept can indeed be reflected in what you look like.

Yes, we are talking about superficialities, qualities that are literally skin-deep. I'm not negating inner beauty because it is usually the driving force of love. But you've first got to catch someone's attention at the beach, at school, or at a business presentation before he or she discovers your deeper qualities.

Psychologists like to remind us that image, confidence, and poise emanate from within. Countless hours and dollars have been spent on pep-talks, motivation, and "life-coaching." I won't disagree entirely with these laudable aims or discourage people from attending seminars, retreats, or any constructive form of group therapy.

But sometimes, behavioral change can take place from the outside in. Consider how putting on Mommy's oversized clothing can transform a young girl into a princess. How about those little boys at a football game who are transformed into future quarterbacks by wearing the uniform or jersey of a sports idol? "Clothes make the man [or woman]" even at a very young age. Does wearing a sexy outfit at a party, at the senior prom or at a club make you act or feel differently?

Therefore, you need work on looking better in two directions. You will never be able to lose weight permanently unless your mindset is changed and you will never improve your self-concept unless you look much more attractive. As you lose weight by following my recommendations, you will also need to change all the other visible components of your image, whether static (in your appearance) or dynamic (in your behavior). Self-improvement must occur in two directions simultaneously, as your healthier body chemistry enhances your looks and your upgraded appearance makes you more desirable and more sociable. To accomplish this, you will learn from an unprecedented team of celebrity consultants whose sole aim is to make your life happier, fuller, and longer.

LET'S GET STARTED

Like Benno Blimpie, the thinner "you" underneath all those layers of padding needs a brief moment in the sun; I have always told my patients not to stare at the bathroom scale but to watch how other people treat them once their appearance changes. I love it when someone reports how shocked their friends are at "The New Me." Admiring looks and flattering comments from other people are much, much more reinforcing, motivating, and stimulating than any bathroom scale reading.

Here's what I'm asking of you: follow my program for only six weeks. Be prepared to take a hard look at yourself and then re-evaluate every aspect of your present image—your weight, your hairstyle, even your fashion sense. Every day for six weeks, you'll have a set of instructions and recommendations on a variety of essential makeover topics—food, fashion, exercise, hairstyle, skincare, self-confidence, and social skills—by an expert in each field. You'll learn a little about psychology too and what makes you the person you are. Errors in thinking will be addressed and debunked. You'll view your food, clothing, and facial appearance in a different way and use the barometer of social approval correctly and skillfully.

I feel sure that even in a short time you'll be amazed at how differently people look at and treat you. At the end of the six weeks, the choice is yours: revert to your old self-abusing habits or continue to grow more and more attractive and desirable. You will also develop a better smile, improve your social skills and become a great conversationalist. And you'll never make Mistake Number One again.

Sound like a good idea? Then let's get started.

I

THE SEVEN AREAS OF IMAGE REINVENTION

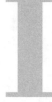he time has arrived for you to reinvent yourself, and you will probably never see yourself the same way again. Change is good, change is exciting, and change is permanent when the rewards are spectacular.

Did you ever fantasize about getting a complete makeover by a team of experts, focusing their attention on every component of your appearance and behavior? Imagine no more: your personal A-list team of image consultants has arrived, preparing to introduce themselves to the new you.

Your image is the sum total of seven components of appearance and behavior:

1. bodily physique
2. weight
3. fashion
4. hair
5. grooming and makeup

6. self-confidence
7. interpersonal skills

Let's start by focusing on what people see when you walk into a room. It's initially a reflection of your physical appearance, which is determined mainly by how you carry your weight and musculature. Since exercise and nutrition are crucial to redefining that infrastructure, who better to guide you on your journey of self-reinvention than a personal trainer to Hollywood stars and a culinary genius whose food is so scrumptious, you'd never guess it was ultra-healthy and calorie-thrifty?

Once you're working on the infrastructure, you'll proceed to studying your "outerwear," the spectacular looks that are defined by the proper hairstyle, clothing, and skincare. At this juncture, your advisors will be among the most experienced and sought-after international experts in their fields, who are now adding you to their esteemed client base.

You'll also be getting a makeover in possibly the most critical aspects of image around, your self-confidence and interpersonal skills. You'll learn from the most seasoned teachers more about yourself and your relationship with the world around you than ever before. You'll become an expert at how to make new relationships that last, as well as becoming the center of attention wherever you go—in short, someone everyone wants to know.

Without further ado, I'd like to present to you the celebrity consultants, who will tell you about themselves, their credentials, their specialties and their basic philosophies. So get ready for your close-up. We're about to start.

1

PARK AVENUE SELF-CONFIDENCE WITH STANLEY KRIPPNER, PH.D.

WHY SELF-CONFIDENCE IS IMPORTANT TO *THE PARK AVENUE DIET*

Self-confidence is the feeling that you can accomplish a task you have undertaken. Truly self-confident people know their strengths and limitations and choose tasks that they know they can complete successfully, as well as embarking on some tasks that challenge them and stretch their capacity to the limit.

Self-confident people avoid self-destructive behavior, procrastination, and anything else that interferes with meeting their goals. Each successful accomplishment boosts their self-confidence. Occasional setbacks and criticism are seen as learning opportunities by self-confident people, not reasons for negative thinking or despair. Self-confident people don't give up. They simply try again.

Self-confidence is not the same as "willpower," which often depends on wishful thinking and fantasy to attain a goal. Self-confidence, in contrast, reflects a realistic assessment of one's capacities. It is built upon emotional reinforcement. Each time you succeed at a task, you feel a sense of accomplishment, and your confidence increases. Each time you make a healthy food choice, you know that you have made the right decision. And this makes it easier to make other healthy choices in the future.

Self-confidence is also not the same as self-esteem. Self-esteem reflects what you think and feel about yourself. Self-confidence reflects what you think and feel about your abilities. It is more accurate to be realistic about your self-confidence because it is built on successful accomplishments—or unsuccessful mishaps as the case may be. Self-esteem does not correlate well with grade point average, money earned per year, or numbers on a bathroom scale. It is more open to self-deception because it might be based on inflated personal myths—statements that constantly run through your mind, reflecting deep-seated feelings and motives—rather than on actual experiences and interactions in the social world. People with high self-esteem think well of themselves. Fine. Great. But you will need more than pie-in-the-sky reassurances that you are a great gal or a honcho hombre to lose weight and keep fit.

Self-confidence should not be confused with self-centeredness. Self-centered people are narcissistic and think only about themselves and their appearance. A self-confident person takes an interest in other people, in community events, in world affairs, and even in politics and spiritual issues. Self-confident people have the inner strength, the convictions, and the resilience to share what they know with others and to do so in a compassionate manner.

Your self-confidence and your self-esteem are aspects of your "self-concept." So is your body image, the inner picture you have painted about your body. Your self-concept is the sum total of all the beliefs, attitudes, and feelings you have about yourself. It reflects the personal myths, both positive and negative, that you hold about your life, your beliefs, and your potentials. As your self-confidence grows, your self-concept is enhanced, your body image improves, and your self-talk helps you maintain your new behaviors. In other words, self-confidence is fundamental to initiating *The Park Avenue Diet* and sticking with it for the rest of your life.

BASIC PRINCIPLES OF SELF-CONFIDENCE

1.

Changing your thoughts and feelings will change your appearance.

Overeating can best be explained by what psychologists call "learning theory," which studies why people think, feel, and behave the way they do. Learning theory explains why people make sensible or foolish choices during their daily activities and how these choices are supported or "reinforced" by praise, gifts, and other rewards. Learning theory also examines how these decisions interact with genetic, hereditary predispositions as well as brain mechanisms.

For example, the brain's prefrontal cortex helps people make decisions. But when it is shut down by stress, anxiety, or dampened self-confidence, impulse behavior—such as binge eating—takes over. Learning theorists show us how bad habits can be modified, changed, or "extinguished" through the use of practical principles that lead to better ways of thinking, feeling, and making decisions.

Poor food choices have become ingrained into many individuals' daily routines, and hard work is needed to undo them. You will need to unlearn and then relearn how, when, what, where, and even why to eat. The payoff is a healthy, joyful lifestyle that will improve your self-confidence, enhance your body image, and change your personal myths for the better.

2.

Your personal failures are linked to your personal myths.

Have you heard of "yo-yo" dieters? They lose several pounds one month, then gain them all back the following month. Many yo-yo dieters end up with a negative self-concept. They harbor feelings of self-loathing, shame, and poor self-esteem because they cannot keep the weight off. And they often smother these negative feelings by eating more food. Of course this makes no sense at all.

But by examining their thoughts and feelings, yo-yo dieters can discover underlying personal myths such as:

> "The thought of losing weight threatens me because I am afraid I will gain it all back."

> "When I lose weight, I feel unprotected; a few extra pounds serve as a buffer between me and the outside world."

> "When I start to lose weight, I realize how much I hate my body, and then I lose interest in anything that would improve it."

Just read and re-read these statements. They are completely irrational and immature, aren't they? If you are afraid that you will gain your weight back, you have lost your motivation to make long-lasting changes. If you think that body flab and fat will protect you from the outside world, you are engaging in "magical thinking," an irrational way of looking at cause and effect. And if your body image is so disagreeable that it generates hate, you need some spiritual direction. In other words, you need to remind yourself that your body was given to you by God, by nature, or by genetics, take your pick. Whatever your world view might be, your body is a sacred gift. And you reject and disparage these types of gifts at your peril.

3.

Each person's healthy eating habits are different, but unhealthy habits are remarkably similar.

Women and men who have learned mature coping skills have developed personal mythologies that help them navigate the turbulent seas of life. But when it comes to unhealthy behavior, there is a much narrower range of personal myths. Health care professionals usually hear the same rationalizations, defenses, and projections so often that they can just about complete their clients' statements for them. So it goes with unhealthy eating habits.

The first step is to replace negative self-talk with positive, life-affirming beliefs, attitudes, and behaviors. Don't think of yourself as a victim. Don't call yourself a "loser." That way of thinking is indulgent and immature. You might have had some tough breaks in life, but so have most of the people you know. If you have not already done so, come to a decision that your days of excuses are over. Old myths die hard. And there may be labor pains associated with giving birth to new myths and new eating habits. But soon you will develop the inner resilience and the external social support that you will integrate into *The Park Avenue Diet*.

Readers of this book will find vastly different ways to implement the suggestions and the advice they will encounter. They will take many different paths to the promised land, making their vision of a new mind and body a reality.

4.

Your mind and body work together.

During the Middle Ages, Europeans decided that thoughts came from above the neck and that feelings came from below the neck. In ancient India, practitioners of yoga did not make a clear-cut division between "mind" and "body." They located both thoughts and feelings in seven "chakras" or energy centers positioned along the spinal cord. The word *yoga* can be translated as *yoke*, a bond between mind and body as well as between humanity and divinity. People who practice yoga are told to eat a sensible diet, practice flexible body postures and deep breathing, and keep mind and body working together. In other words, yoga has many of the basic principles as *The Park Avenue Diet*. More specifically, self-confidence is an example of a trait that yokes body and mind, feelings and thoughts, intellect and emotion. Most emotions are experiences and are communicated nonverbally, so you can't depend on words alone to change your personal myths. Don't let your thoughts take over your emotions, and don't let your moods kidnap your thoughts. Pull your resources together.

5.

Overeating is an equal opportunity bad habit.

Don't allow yourself to think, "Weight loss is only important for people who have a public image to maintain." You have a public, too—a public of friends, families, and co-workers. If you look good at family events, social gatherings, and office parties, you will influence the social dynamics of the event. Most people will feel more at ease with you, will want to spend more time in your company, and even compliment you. You'll feel more self-confident, too. And every time someone compliments you, this reinforcement will help you to keep the weight off and look good or even better than ever.

6.

Mistaken perceptions can lead to overeating.

Many psychologists study perception—vision, hearing, taste, touch, and smell—and how perception affects eating habits. People eat less and enjoy food more when focusing on the sight, taste, texture, and smell of every delicious bite. But perception can also deceive you. If you choose a large plate when you go through a buffet, you will put more food on it than if you choose a small plate. You might think you are taking the same amount, but your perceptions have fooled you because of the size of the plate.

The same principle holds for what you drink. Thus, at a party or a buffet, choose the smallest possible plate and glass to ensure moderation and sociability. You'll be perceived differently as well, as people focus on your opinions, outfit, or sociability, not on your eating habits.

7.

Learn to make decisions on your own.

Some individuals are not especially influenced by their environment or their circle of friends. Others are more easily influenced by people around them. They easily succumb to such suggestions as "Let's go out and have a pizza," or, "How about joining us for a beer?"

These people typically have a difficult time losing weight and keeping weight off. They often eat when they are not hungry but when they are "cued in" by the people around them. Other cues include the color of the plates and dishes, the attractiveness of the way a food is presented or packaged, various food shapes and food smells, even the distance between them and the refrigerator or the food cupboard.

If you think that you are easily influenced by others, establish a daily routine around eating and do not deviate from it. Don't let distractions disrupt that routine. This discipline is part of the self-regulation that will keep you looking good and feeling healthy.

Remember that new healthy eating habits are grounded in the creation of new neural networks in your brain. You strengthen these networks every time you put a sensible routine into practice. Changing poor eating habits involves breaking up other neural networks. In other words, following the *The Park Avenue Diet* will not only change your appearance, it will change your brain.

8.

A comprehensive approach to weight loss is the best approach.

We will be doing several exercises that apply learning theory to improving your social skills and shared interactions. This may seem a radical way to lose weight. Why not just eat sensibly, make some resolutions, and watch the scale every day? *The Park Avenue Diet* wants you to keep the weight off once you have shed those extra pounds. Willpower is rarely successful because it does not strike at the irrational thinking and childish personal myths that underlie poor eating habits. When you are setting goals, make the goals realistic. When you make affirmations, don't set the bar too high. Learning theory tells us that success is important for making long-lasting changes. Success enhances self-confidence. Failure undermines it.

When your friends start telling you that you are looking great, that you are dressing better, and that you surprise them with your new charm and charisma, the feedback will enhance your self-confidence and do more to keep you on track than all the scales and resolutions in the world. This positive reinforcement will give you the feeling of accomplishment that underlies the motivation you need to make *The Park Avenue Diet* a permanent part of your life.

9.

Spiritual attitudes play an important role in developing self-confidence.

Many people who have successfully and permanently lost weight give credit to their spirituality. More than one successful dieter has said: "I was having trouble sticking to my diet when I realized that I was doing a great disservice to God, my Creator. God gave me life, my body, and my capacity for organizing that life and regulating that body. Once I had this spiritual awakening, it was easy for me to shed pounds, to eat sensibly, to exercise, to meditate, and to examine all of my thoughts and feelings to see if they were supporting my new self-concept."

This is an example of "insight learning," a change in behavior in which a sudden insight, often called an "intuition," produces a rapid advance toward a goal. Insight learning often arrives through dreams, through prayer, through meditation, through "flow" experiences, or simply after all intellectual approaches to solving a problem have failed.

10.

Make sure you have a solid support group.

You are fortunate if you have a social support group that endorses your adherence to *The Park Avenue Diet*. But what if you are surrounded by "enablers" who think they are "taking care" of you by reinforcing unhealthy food choices?

These enablers may be parents who encourage overeating in the name of comfort and nurturance. They may be spouses who believe that being a provider means putting huge amounts of food in front of their family. They may say things like:

> "I really don't agree with your brother when he says that you have put on weight. You look just fine to me."

> "What's wrong with indulging in a second dessert? You work hard and you deserve some pleasure."

"Let's not talk about unpleasant topics tonight. Instead,
let go to the pizzeria and have ourselves a feast."

Become aware of enablers and listen critically to the personal and family myths that they want you to accept. For the most part, enablers are not nasty people. They mean well, but the road to obesity is often paved with good intentions. Think through their advice and the impact it would make on your appearance if you followed it.

ASSESSING YOUR SELF-CONFIDENCE

Self-confidence is a trait that allows people to have positive yet realistic views of themselves, their lives, and their abilities. Self-confident people trust their capacities, have a general sense of control, and believe that, in most situations, they will be able to accomplish what they expect to do. Even when some of their expectations are not met, they continue to maintain positive feelings about themselves, and learn from their setbacks.

People who lack self-confidence depend excessively on other peoples' approval and avoid taking risks because they are afraid of failure. They often are excessively self-critical and ignore compliments.

You can take this simple test to determine your level of self-confidence. Answer Yes or No to the following statements:

1. I am willing to risk the disapproval of other people if I really believe in what I am doing.
2. It is important for me to conform to other peoples' standards so that they will accept me.
3. My expectations are realistic; I realize that I can not be an expert in everything.
4. I am very critical of myself, but I make so many mistakes that I really don't deserve praise from myself or others.
5. My friends' comments are more important than my own beliefs about my abilities.

6. I feel that I must always have love and approval of each significant person in my life.
7. I believe that I am a worthy person, even though I am not perfect.
8. I can learn from my past accomplishments but I can also learn from my failures and setbacks.
9. I must always be on guard because potential disaster looms around every corner.
10. Something is wrong with me if I can not follow a conversation when I am with strangers.
11. I approach new experiences to learn rather than as an occasion to win something.
12. I realize that I cannot do everything perfectly, but I can enjoy difficult tasks anyway.

Give yourself one point for each question if you answered YES to items 1, 3, 7, 8, 11, 12.

Give yourself one point for each questions if you answered NO to items 2, 4, 5, 6, 9, and 10.

Each of these statements is a personal myth. As you can see, some myths are positive and some are negative. Some help us develop self-confidence while others undermine it.

The higher your score, the more likely it is that self-confidence will be your ally in losing weight and upgrading your image.

PARK AVENUE DINING WITH CHEF MARIE-ANNICK COURTIER

ABOUT CHEF MARIE-ANNICK COURTIER

Chef Marie-Annick Courtier, born and raised in Paris, has mastered the culinary arts through experience and education in diverse aspects of her field. Drawing upon her early triumphs as a sports champion, she has made health consciousness a part of her career, academic achievements, business projects, and personal mission.

One of very few gourmet chefs to hold degrees in both food preparation and physical education, she has focused her attention and insights on proper nutrition for children, adults, and families. An author, lecturer, athletic coach, teacher, and highly successful caterer, Chef Marie has also started her own personal fitness chef program, a perfect representation of the philosophy of "sound mind, sound body." Her acclaimed recipes for *The Saint Tropez Diet* (Hatherleigh, 2006) translate the Mediterranean diet into extraordinarily healthy meals that are as easy to prepare as they are elegant and flavorful.

With a truly comprehensive approach to fine dining and devotion to the health and longevity of her clients, colleagues, and students, Chef Marie is the ideal culinary expert for readers of *The Park Avenue Diet*.

WHY HEALTHY DINING IS IMPORTANT TO *THE PARK AVENUE DIET*

My interest in nutrition began very early in life. I was a table tennis champion when I was young and realized as a teenager that eating right influenced my performance. Eventually I pursued a career in the culinary world, but what I learned from sports carried over well to cooking school.

My mentor and supervisor in cooking school was Chef Al, a tutor who developed my interest in healthy dining, which has several components. First, choose fresh, natural ingredients and emphasize their flavor with simplicity: using the fewest possible ingredients guarantees a more flavorful meal. Flavor, by the way, is a beautiful gift from nature. Moreover, when you use fewer and more distinctive flavors, you actually minimize cooking time.

Second, healthy dining depends on the quantity of food on the table. A basic problem in the United States is that our meals are inappropriately oversized. In our fast-paced society, the speed of eating has become so much more important than the contents of the meal that we often forget to listen to our body's signals when we've had enough.

Third, healthy dining focuses on the pleasure of eating and then on our nutritional needs. Having a meal is more than simply "fueling up" your body. The French "live for eating," meaning that eating and socializing around food are priorities. Italy, Spain, and Greece are other countries I enjoy visiting, places where food is also an important part of life.

When I first came to the United States in 1977, it was a bit that way here. But over the years, productivity and money have taken over. This may be one of the causes of the obesity epidemic in this country.

Another possible explanation is that Americans may actually have too much "nutritional" information bombarding them—it's now just "background noise." Most Americans don't know what to believe. In France, you will rarely hear such information in the media, nor will people discuss it. Why? Because it is taught at an early age and re-emphasized through everyday meal rituals. People rely on those structures and don't even think of questioning them.

Too often, in the United States, we produce foods that will last forever on the shelf, not foods that reflect a love of life. This is highly unnatural, and the results are readily seen on overweight bodies. Added sugar, salt, and other preservatives and additives dull our taste buds and contribute to diabetes, heart disease, and a host of other health problems.

In contrast, growing up in France provided me with an early education in the importance of nutrition, personal appearance, and self-respect. French women can develop weight problems just like anyone else in the world, but we have learned to look at ourselves objectively. If we overindulge, we make up for it with extra exercise, including daily activities such as walking to school with our children.

Did you know that a basic education in France includes a detailed study of all the five senses? My senses of taste and smell are extremely developed. I can tell you most of the ingredients of a particular dish when I walk past a store or restaurant. It may take a while to appreciate how important this approach to food is, but a new world will open up to you. When you drink wine, for instance, don't gulp it down like water; feel it, smell it, and savor it as a sensual pleasure of the highest order.

The pleasure of creating and exploring flavors is part of how we make life worth living. Additionally, there is a therapeutic and a social side to cooking and eating, as we enjoy sharing our time and our creations with others. Don't cook alone. Share the experience: It's quality time for friends and family.

Life is full of sensory experiences: take the time to hear, see, smell, touch, and taste things. These sensory experiences will reach your soul, and then you will live your life full of pleasure, beauty, and good health—and you will reach your healthy weight.

BASIC PRINCIPLES OF HEALTHY DINING

1. Understand your emotions and how they influence your eating habits and therefore your lifestyle.
2. Educate your senses for tasting food and developing healthy habits.
3. Learn what is the right amount of food for your daily bodily needs.
4. Choose superior quality ingredients from the most natural sources.
5. Learn healthy cooking techniques.
6. Be adventurous in cooking and in life.
7. Share your passion for fine dining with others.
8. Be sure to have sharp knives and paring knives for proper food preparation.
9. Take inventory frequently of your pots and pans. Calphalon stainless steel or aluminum pans are the best: they are heavy on the bottom and cook evenly on the entire surface. Teflon is great for low-fat cooking.
10. Live for healthy, pleasurable eating.

SELF-ASSESSMENT OF DINING HABITS

1. Salt is a necessary addition to every food served on my plate.
2. Trans fats are healthy components of food that help to lower cholesterol.
3. Complex carbohydrates enter the bloodstream more gradually and stabilize blood sugar levels more effectively than simple carbohydrates.
4. Legumes are a good source of protein and fiber.
5. The deeper the color of fruits and vegetables, the lower the antioxidant activity.
6. Regular consumption of nuts such as walnuts, almonds, or hazelnuts may reduce the risk of developing diabetes and heart disease.
7. Grilled or broiled items are often a healthier choice on a restaurant menu.
8. A small baked potato can be a healthier choice than fries.
9. It does not matter which salad dressing I use, since it adds few calories.
10. Yogurt contains live bacterial cultures that are good for you.
11. Salad bars are a great choice for eating out.
12. Fruits and honey are a good source of sweeteners.

Answers:

1. False. Many prepared foods already contain more salt than your body needs.
2. False. Trans fats are unhealthy because they raise LDL ("bad") cholesterol and lower HDL ("good") cholesterol levels, increasing the risk of coronary artery disease.
3. True.
4. True. Legumes such as peas, lentils, beans, and soybeans are a great source of protein.
5. False.
6. True.
7. True. However, be aware of rich fatty sauces served on the side. Inquire if the chef can baste the food with canola or olive oil rather than clarified butter (if not advertised). Ask for grilled or steamed vegetables, not fries.

8. True. The use of butter, sour cream, cheese, or bacon as toppings is what will make this choice unhealthy. Mix in a little olive oil and fresh herbs instead.

9. False. Some dressings contains high amount of fat, sodium, and calories. Tossing a little lemon/orange juice, oil and vinegar, or a flavorful herbed vinaigrette with the lettuce or salad before plating will spread the dressing evenly, limiting its quantity and therefore calories.

10. True. They contain beneficial bacteria that fight intestinal pathogens. Yogurt is also a good source of calcium.

11. False. Many people have a tendency to eat more calories from a salad bar than from a fixed menu.

12. True.

PARK AVENUE FITNESS WITH BERNADETTE PENOTTI

ABOUT BERNADETTE PENOTTI

Bernadette Penotti has been a celebrity personal trainer, exercise expert, and glamorous actor for many years, treasured by her clients and associates for her dynamic workout, warmth, spirituality and ebullient personality. She has trained Hollywood stars such as Kate Beckinsale, Melanie Griffith, and many other notables (including Dr. Stuart Fischer) while performing in *The Sopranos*, *Law & Order*, *Kiss of Death*, *Regarding Henry*, and *No Way Home*. She will also debut in her own radio interview show, co-starring the distinguished actor/producer Fisher Stevens, with guests stars from the A-list of the entertainment world. When your business associates and colleagues include Bruce Willis, Gary Oldman, Sean Connery, Tim Roth, Harrison Ford and James Gandolfini, only the most spectacular looks will do!

Ms. Penotti's comprehensive approach to fitness and her devotion to the health and happiness of her clients make her the ideal choice as the exercise expert for *The Park Avenue Diet*.

WHY FITNESS IS IMPORTANT TO
THE PARK AVENUE DIET

I started out with an average body—kind of a "ruler" shape with large breasts. There were stages when I was very slim and those where "I packed it on." In my mid-20s after several years of being a fitness professional, mostly teaching step aerobics, I rediscovered weight training. I had been there before, having five brothers and a very athletic dad who had me lifting weights in the garage with them as we were growing up—I did everything to keep up! Back in the gym, I first experimented with machines and barbells for my lower body—leg presses, hamstring curls, and lunges. There was an immediate improvement, especially in my tush, which immediately looked rounder and firmer.

I was hooked! I learned many more exercises for my lower body and started to train my upper body as well. It was like KAPOW! I went from a ruler to "curves in all the right places" with very little body fat. At the time I was working as an actress in New York City, so it helped to look good. In a very short time, I was hired to play roles on top TV shows including *Law & Order, Sex and the City, As the World Turns,* and *The Sopranos.*

Most of the roles had me playing women who were considered to be sexy, exotic, or bombshell types. It was fun, and my confidence was growing too. I knew a lot of it had to do with my new figure. In order to keep it, I devised a workout that could be done anywhere—at home, on my parents' living room floor, on the film set, or even in my miniscule room in the movie-set trailer or "honey wagon."

I'd enroll whoever was around to join me, and we'd get in shape in between takes. It was tricky not to mess up my costume or hair, but I was determined to squeeze my workout into the often 12- to 15-hour workdays. On the grip truck (the truck that holds film equipment), there was often a bar across the back of the truck. I'd use it to do pull ups, or I'd do pushups with the Teamsters, squats with the lead actress, and lunges with anyone else. I took my portable training system everywhere.

Eventually, I became a personal trainer to a number of great actors and film executives, including Jake Weber, Jamie-Lynn Sigler, Joe Bob Briggs and Kathrine Narducci. My specialty: getting my clients in great shape safely in the shortest amount of time. No equipment required—or we'd just use simple dumbbells and a bench—and an ample sprinkling of fun. To this day I especially enjoy helping women lose weight and sculpt their bodies beautiful.

Over the years I have honed my approach to further assist my time-challenged clients. I began to train them using short, intense workouts that combined cardio (or aerobic training) with weight training. Also known as interval training, this series of upper and lower body exercises using compound movements challenges the heart, burns calories, and saves a lot of time. Fat disappears, lean muscles show up, digestion improves, joint pain diminishes, bone density increases, blood pressure goes down, and cholesterol improves. Good stuff! And the best part: the whole session takes only 20 to 30 minutes, which we do three times a week. That's it! When you have time, other practices such as yoga, Pilates, or Tai Chi are beneficial and complementary.

In just a few weeks, with three 30-minute sessions per week combined with good nutrition and proper rest, my clients would see a big change in their health, body composition, posture, and overall attractiveness. It's definitely an "inside-out, outside-in" proposition, as Dr Fischer so aptly puts it...it's exciting and it's 100% possible for you too!

BASIC PRINCIPLES OF FITNESS

1.

There are four essential components to a great fitness program: aerobic training, resistance training, nutrition, and rest and recovery.

- **Aerobic training,** better known as "cardio" because it is defined as an elevation of the heart rate that is steadily maintained for at least 20 minutes. You can calculate your maximal heart rate, the fastest it can beat in one minute in a healthy, productive manner, by subtracting your age from 220.
- **Resistance training (sometimes called strength training, or anaerobic training),** namely challenging your muscles so they will become stronger and more functional. You can accomplish this with weights, bands, cables, and even your own body weight. Whatever means you use, here's the deal: you've got to "press" to be your best.
- **Nutrition,** the proper way to feed and nurture your attractive new physique.
- **Rest and recovery,** to make your workouts more effective.

2.

Exercise, like all the important things in life, requires commitment.

Start slowly and intensify gradually: our *Park Avenue Diet* exercise regimen will be constructed in a way that begins relatively easily. Yet, by the conclusion, you will have mastered an excellent workout—you'll see how very soon. Pick a time, a place, and a healthy snack . . . and get to it. Mornings are the best time: putting it off until the afternoon usually becomes skipping it.

3.

Basic exercises done with perfect form will be the foundation of your workout.

This goes for those new to exercise, the vets, and the elite. Whether you are 17 or 70 years of age there are the "staple" or core movements that, done correctly, will support every body (i.e. squats, lunges, pushups, shoulder presses).

4.

Compound movements—movements that use many muscle groups at the same time—rock big time!

A good example is the "squat" which uses virtually every muscle in the lower body. Compound movements are the king of burning calories and melting fat— which will allow us to see your sexy, gorgeous muscles underneath!

5.

For best results and time management, do "interval training."

Alternate short bursts of high-intensity exercises with a short recovery period. Moving quickly from one strength-training exercise to another will simultaneously build muscle and elevate heart rate—more "bang for the buck" as you get your aerobic and anaerobic components fulfilled at the same time.

6.

You must use a full range of motion for your muscles to grow and strengthen properly—as well as to get a thorough stretch.

Though we will move from one exercise to another quickly—30 to 60 seconds between sets—we will perform each individual exercise slowly and thoughtfully.

Slow movements recruit more muscle fiber. Therefore, a good rule of thumb for each exercise repetition is 2 counts on the way up, and 4 counts on the way down.

7.

Breathe, Breathe, Breathe!

The basic idea is to keep breathing throughout each exercise—exhaling (breathing out) on the exertion (when standing up from a squat) and inhaling as you release (as you sit down into the squat). Exercise is a heightened form of normal movement, needing more blood flow, warmth, and oxygen.

8.

Use the beneficial "push/pull" sequence.

If you do a movement where you are "pushing or pressing" (like a push-up or shoulder press) it's best to follow that with a "pulling" movement (like bent-over rows or lat pull-downs). This gives a balanced approach to the way the muscles are used and feels great, too!

9.

Engage your mind in the workout.

Showing up 100% and focusing on the movements, as opposed to "phoning it in" builds more muscle fibers: "What you focus on grows."

10.

Make sure to get a solid night's sleep after each day's training.

It is also crucial to give your body plenty of hydration from pure water, fresh fruits, and veggies to rejuvenate your entire system.

SELF-ASSESSMENT OF POSTURE

I'm sure that you know how much you weigh and it's just as easy to measure your height (for extra credit, you may also have calculated your Body Mass Index). Let's disregard them all for now and do a very simple experiment to assess your posture, an important component of physical appearance.

Take a piece of paper and turn it sideways so you're looking directly at the longer edge. This is going to represent your spine. Bring the top and bottom of the piece of paper slightly closer together; the piece of paper will appear to 'bulge' in the middle.

Now it's your turn to replicate this fascinating phenomenon. Stand in front of a full-length mirror and turn sideways. Pretend that you are a tired commuter coming home from work after a two-hour train ride; your shoulders are sinking, your spine is collapsing due to exhaustion, and perhaps you're even leaning slightly forward.

Take a look at your belly; it's more prominent and globular, and not because you've just eaten a large pizza. Just like the restructuring of that two-dimensional piece of paper, your midriff bulges from the artificial shortening of your spinal column. In other words, poor posture can make you look fatter than you are.

Pick a nice, clean area of your home, and lie down on your back. Make sure that virtually your entire spine is in contact with the floor. Imagine that your body is being stretched out, with your head as far "north" and your heels as far "south" as possible.

Your body has just attained its maximal length (and you will need to develop the musculature to keep it this way under normal circumstances). What happened to your abdomen? It's somewhat smaller, and not merely because of gravitational forces. Think of the "remolding" of that piece of paper.

Now, stand up and try again to assume these two different body shapes, slumped over and as tall as possible. Better posture will help you look thinner and healthier in ways that hundreds of sit-ups won't.

Today, check yourself every few hours in a mirror, wherever you are. Is your spine collapsing? Are you as fully elongated as when you were stretched out on your living room floor? When you get home, remind yourself how it feels by another session of this exercise. Your body will eventually be extremely grateful.

PARK AVENUE FASHION
WITH HELENE HELLSTEN

WHY FASHION IS IMPORTANT TO
THE PARK AVENUE DIET

When you walk into a room, everyone inside will spend about three seconds formulating an overall impression of you, even before a word is said, even if you're a total stranger. Put another way, "You only have one chance to make a good first impression." A great sense of humor, dazzling business skills, or knowing the latest sports scores—no one will be able to see these qualities initially. What they will see is how you look.

Looking great is a combination of many different elements, all of which you'll be addressing in due course. And that's especially true when it comes to what you wear. Choosing the right outfit, caring for your clothing, re-evaluating the contents of your closets, keeping up with the latest styles—all are important ways to make sure that you look terrific throughout the day, wherever you go, whatever social or business situations you find yourself in.

Looking good is part of one's entire day. At the gym, or in the company of very close friends, or even alone, make the effort to dress with taste and self-awareness. There's no moment where sloppiness or laxity should creep in. It's true that different situations require different strategies: work versus an evening on the town, for example. Part of the learning curve will involve your observations of others. But our approach will hold true for any budget level, encompassing clothing style, color, and texture.

The better you look, the more confident you feel—and the more confident you feel, the more carefully you'll select your outfits for the day. Our complex lives and relationships depend on self-confidence, and a lack of self-confidence sends the wrong message to the social world around us.

Caring about others must come from within, and this must be reflected in self-care as well. One's self-confidence should be unshakable, steadfast, and almost contagious, not overemphasized or overstated. And speaking about overstatement—you might think that, as an international fashion consultant, I prefer complex and intricate combinations of clothing. On the contrary; I favor simplicity and focus to excessive adornment and overdressing.

Just as a new, more slender "you" makes you happier and prouder, you can develop a new comfort zone by learning how to choose the right fashions and accessories. I want you to feel more comfortable too and to make these choices almost effortlessly and even instinctively, once you've learned the basic rules of my philosophy. Besides, looking good (and learning how to) is lots of fun. The "new you" will still be the same person, but you will have a new wardrobe—in fact, an entire lifestyle—that will make you a more confident and attractive person who will make a wonderful impression on everyone.

BASIC PRINCIPLES OF FASHION

I'd like to share with you some of my most important principles of dressing well, concepts that are true whether I'm focusing on an individual's appearance or reviewing an entire catalogue for a large department store.

1.

First impressions are made in three seconds!

Have you ever heard the expressions "the dress is wearing her" or "he's only a suit"? It simply means that if you see clothes before you notice the people wearing them, they're probably overdressed or bizarrely decked out.

Along these lines, when putting together an outfit, you should always aim for style, not drama. Just remember that no matter what you wear, it must be clean and unwrinkled.

2.

Start studying fashion magazines.

Don't expect to master all the principles of fashion in a few days. You need some time to decide on and develop a new style for yourself.

One tip I find extremely valuable is to buy magazines that feature a lifestyle and fashion slant closest to your personal ideal. The publications could range from those that deal with haute couture to fitness. It all depends on the setting that seems most natural to you. Study the attire that is being featured, then imagine yourself in that environment, appropriately clad.

3.

Make colors and shapes work for you.

In the early days of *The Park Avenue Diet,* here are some basic rules to follow (as you grow more confident in your fashion choices, you'll learn how to vary these a little):

- Choose outfits organized around a single color—they're slimming.
- No big patterns, please—unless you're trying to look like a billboard.

- Contrary to what you've always been told, loose-fitting clothes do *not* make you look thinner. Fitted outfits do the trick.
- No scoop necks—ever. They add an appearance of fullness to the face, neck and shoulders.

4.

Have your size re-evaluated at every shopping opportunity.

Get to know which size is what and which matches best with your shape and stature. Petite, women's, or ladies'? For men it's trial and error. Brands from Italy tend to have smaller sizes, but if you're very tall, go for German brands.

5.

Charity begins in your closet.

Make it a habit to do a yearly wardrobe inventory. Even if clothes have sentimental value, when they no longer fit and/or look out of style, say goodbye to them, pack them up and send them to a charity where they will make a positive difference in the lives of those less fortunate than you.

6.

Less is definitely more.

Here are the three undisputed categories of clothes that must go:

- Pieces that look worn out and are verging on shabby.
- Clothes that age you like last season's butterfly pants.
- Styles you had to have five years ago and haven't worn since.

7.

Simplicity is a virtue.

Self-confidence in your clothing style translates into well-selected and simple outfits, whether you travel light or with lots of stuff. The trick is to look like you made no effort to dress.

8.

Be realistic about sizes, especially online.

Mail order and shopping on the Internet is great and ultra-convenient, but even when a measurement table is included, it's often hard to select the size that will fit you perfectly. Some companies size down, some size up; and. European sizes differ from American sizes. Since you're the only judge of how you look, it's best to try things on.

Use mail order or computer clothes selection only if you're the type of person who will go to the trouble of sending it back if it's not right for you. Otherwise, forget it!

9.

Clothing needs to fit perfectly.

As you slim down to a smaller size, you have to check your wardrobe often to see how the clothes you used to wear fit you now. Always make sure you have a great fit. When a piece of clothing becomes hopelessly too big, get rid of it.

10.

Quality is important.

Never compromise on quality. Ever. Upscale designs and fabrics are more costly for a reason—they look, fit, and wear better. The last thing you want is to wear a blazer that looks like the upholstery in a used car. Keep abreast of holiday and seasonal sales at shops and department stores. You can pick up classic pieces at an affordable price.

10 RULES FOR DETERMINING WHETHER OR NOT YOU'RE OVERDRESSED OR UNDERDRESSED

First check the venue. Is it a business meeting? Is the dress code casual or formal? In general it is as bad to be overdressed as underdressed. But the lesser of two evils is to be overdressed.

Nothing is as important as the impression you give. For women it is always safe to have a pair of good quality black pants with a white shirt and a nice light wool or cotton blazer. Dress it up with scarves and high heels. Dress it down with flat shoes and fun custom jewelery. Sometimes I carry high heels and a nice silk scarf. If I realize I have misunderstood the occasion I change in the restroom.

Men can do the same: always have a silk tie with you if you need to change from casual to dressed up. If during a business meeting, lunch, or dinner some of the men take off their jackets you can do the same.

1. Check out the environment beforehand—bar, office, restaurant. Is it an upscale place? Check the website. What time of the day and week is it? Business casual is usually okay for a Friday and weekends.

2. When you travel a lot you realize that there are different traditions in different countries, even in different parts of a country. I usually call the hotel where I am staying to check temperature and dress code in general.

3. It is very telling when you see the CEO wearing shoes without socks at a meeting. This happens frequently in the music industry. If you are participating in meeting with accountants, however, dress accordingly—i.e., low-key and safe.

4. When you realize that people are looking over your shoulder and back you have probably fooled around with distracting patterns or too many accessories. For men, this is usually a terrible tie; for women, earrings and clicking bracelets. Then you know you are overdressed. Try to dismantle the damage ASAP.

5. When you feel confident, you know you have dressed according to the code. People listen and talk to you, not your shell.

6. It is not okay to dress haphazardly when out in public. If you visit a church, a supermarket, or the gym, try to step into something that will be appropriate in each place.

7. If other people seem uncomfortable, it's a possible sign that something is wrong with your appearance. Anything from marmalade stains to overpowering clothes may

result in interpersonal distress. Remember to check the mirror.

8. Sometimes it is impossible even for the most organized of us to leave a great impression. Maybe the dry cleaner fooled around with your garments or your airline made sure your bag never arrived. Try to stay calm. Buy a tie or a scarf, and just try to be yourself.

9. New outfits are sometimes scary. You have to break them in and wear them on different occasions to figure out where they work the best. Do this slowly.

10. Ask sales people or personal shoppers for advice. This is the best advice always! Local knowledge is king.

10 RULES FOR CHOOSING THE RIGHT COLORS FOR YOURSELF IN CLOTHING

1. For business occasions always wear black, dark blue, and white.

2. It is important to remember your complexion, hair color, eye color, and even age whether you like it or not. Soft colors will make you look more subdued.

3. Do you want to express yourself as serious or funny? Some people love bright colors and depending on the climate (namely, the tropics or the beach), it might be okay. But if you don't work in a fast food restaurant, why attract attention to a bright outfit instead of yourself?

To choose the right color you also have to determine at what time the occasion takes place, particularly if it is an evening event. Go with solid basics and add a splash of color complementing your eyes (see the chart below). Men, a tie in a shade within the color group will be perfect. Always solid, please! Women, try a belt, a shawl, a bag, or earrings. Eveningwear should be simple, not excessive.

Eye Color	Accessory Color
green	intense pink
blue	green
brown	orange
gray	strong blue
black	yellow

4. When you're tired or stressed out, you have to be extra picky about the colors you wear because they will make you or break you. Always try out a color in the light you are going to wear it in. Even swim trousers or bathing suits look terrible in the wrong light. Ask your sales associate to follow you on the street to take a look at the true color. White in any shade will always help you to look your best.

5. When you go from a business meeting to a party, make sure you only add one color so you don't have to change everything. Start with black and white and add some color that you feel comfortable in.

6. Ask experienced sales people what color they recommend. Trust them. You will soon see a pattern for yourself. Some colors are too dramatic for most occasions. I would like most of us not to wear chartreuse, green, neon yellow, or neon pink. Orange is tricky because it's nice for casual occasions but is so wrong for business occasions. You don't want to look like an escaped prisoner.

7. Gray is always a safety blanket but too much can age you dramatically—try to mix it with cream or white.

8. Color mixes in patterns can be fantastic or totally catastrophic. The Bahamas shirt is a no-no at the office, as is a shirt with polka dots—always. We are not dalmatians.

9. Think about textures and materials as well as colors. To mix different shades of cream in different materials, such as wool, silk, cotton, is usually fantastic. Men's suits in subtle wool prints from the same color family are always a safe bet.

10. Your color preference is a bit like eating. If you like toma-
    toes you like them red and ripe. Choosing fruits by their
    color is a part of learning how to shop. But sometimes we
    get into a pattern when we don't try new things and that's
    too bad. This is a habit and a trap that many people fall
    into. Out of routine, they shop and eat the same thing,
    every day, all month, and year-round. Needless to say,
    the right color within a color family can enhance your
    appearance a lot.

SELF-ASSESSMENT OF FASHION

Rather than have a self-assessment quiz about your knowledge of fashion,
let's take inventory of your clothing closets to see if you have all the necessary elements to put together great outfits for multiple different occasions.
Here is a checklist of leisure, formal, professional, sports, and shoe wardrobes
for men and women.

LEISURE WARDROBE

Men	Women
jeans – 2	jeans – 3
khakis – 2	khakis – 2
shorts – 3	shorts – 2
T-shirts – 10	T-shirts – 15
polo shirts – 5	polo shirts – 5
shirts, casual – 5	shirts, business plain – 5
	shirts, business with details – 5
	shirts, casual – 5
socks – 15	socks – 15
sweatshirts – 5	sweatshirts – 5
knits – 3	knits – 6
jacket – 3	jacket – 3
blazer – 1 blue	skirts – 3
	tops, form-fitting basic – 5
	tops, "fluid" or "flowing" fabric – 5
	casual dress – 3

PROFESSIONAL/FORMAL WARDROBE

Whether you're dressing for a formal occasion or a business meeting, consider the following suggestions of items to own:

Men	Women
suit – 1	pants suit – 1
shirts, business – 10	little black cocktail dress – 2
black tie – 1	long dress – 1
coat – 1	coat – 2
knits, pullover of good quality in a dark color – 1	knits, basic (preferably cashmere wrap or wool) – 1
	knits, dressy (preferably cardigan with nice buttons) –1

If you don't go black tie often, there's no need to buy a tuxedo. Rent one.

SHOE INVENTORY

Men	Women
sneakers – 3	sneakers – 3
leather boots – 1	leather boots – 2
leather shoes – 3	flats – 2
	high heels – 2
rain and snow boots – 1	rain and snow boots – 1
loafers – 2	loafers – 1
sandals – 0!!	sandals, flats – 2
	high heels – 2
flip-flops – 1	flip-flops – 3

You should own at least one pair of black and one pair of brown shoes—which are almost universally appropriate for both sexes. Women, if I were you, I'd leave white shoes for the bride—they're distracting on anybody else. And remember, whether you're a man or a woman, if your feet are going to be exposed in sandals or flip-flops, a pedicure is a must, not a luxury.

SPORTS CLOTHES

golf – 2 sets

ski – 1 sets

tennis – 3 sets

hikes – 2 sets

surf – 2 sets

yoga – 2 sets

aerobics – 2 sets

biking – 2 sets

power walks – 2 sets

swimming – 3 sets

PARK AVENUE COIFFEUR
WITH JOEL WARREN

ABOUT JOEL WARREN

A native New Yorker, **Joel Warren** grew up in the capital of fashion and beauty. He began styling hair in his early twenties, and while working at several salons, Joel found color to be his true calling. In 1989 he joined with the superlative stylist Edward Tricomi to launch the first Warren-Tricomi Salon, and their spectacular success and thrilled patrons have helped them expand to Greenwich, Los Angeles, and the Hamptons.

An empathetic and gifted artist, Joel constantly works with top models, socialites and celebrities, such as Ivanka Trump, Jessica Alba, Molly Sims, Kate Beckinsale, Anna Paquin, Paulina Porizkova, Rachel Hunter, Amanda Hearst, and Vanessa Haydon. His interest in the care and health of hair reflects his deep dedication to a client's overall sense of beauty and happiness. There is no doubt that he is the ideal expert in his field to be a celebrity consultant for *The Park Avenue Diet*.

WHY YOUR COIFFEUR IS IMPORTANT TO
THE PARK AVENUE DIET

People sometimes ask me how I got interested in my chosen profession. Actually, my original fascination was with beauty, particularly as reflected in the world of the arts. I enjoyed painting as a child and also became proficient in arts and crafts. Somehow I got drawn into doing hair. Needless to say, for me and my clients, creating the right look requires an artistic sensibility, not just manual dexterity.

Like almost everyone else, I have had a wide variety of hairstyles. All reflected my self-image at the time and, of course, mirrored the current social, cultural, and even political trends. In the 1960s and 1970s, you would have seen me with a ponytail or a shaved head—dramatically different styles, to say the least.

My hairstyle evolved in the process, as it should with everyone. A famous principle of physics states that "the only thing constant is change" and that is certainly true of our hair as we journey through life.

Besides needing to reflect our changing features, hairstyles reflect our changing world. Looks are always in evolution, often quite rapidly, and it's important to keep up with the times. Of course, certain styles can be considered classic: the lacquered look of the 1940s movie stars such as Cary Grant and Tyrone Power has been "borrowed" by modern celebrities like George Clooney and Brad Pitt, particularly at gala events.

Your hairstyle says a lot about you. But it does so in conjunction with many other visible "statements," all of which need to work in harmony. Your overall appearance can be broken down into several elements: hair, makeup, clothing, and jewelry. You cannot neglect one and overemphasize the others. Even when I am asked what's the first thing I notice in someone's hairstyle, my answer depends on the balance achieved with those other elements of appearance.

Are most people good judges of how their hair should look? For the most part I would say "yes." But can they do it for themselves? Only to a certain level. In a restaurant you are able to make your food choices from a wide variety of possibilities, but a culinary critic might get you to try something new that you really enjoy. You can go to a department store and choose new clothing, but a fashion designer might select an even more stunning outfit. Similarly, you might know how to make your hair look good, but it usually takes expert help to make it fabulous.

There's an interesting interplay between how our hair looks and how we perceive ourselves. It's really a two-way street, as appearance affects our inner thoughts while our self-image determines how we should look. A new hair color or style can change our mood, our self-confidence, and even our behavior with others. I see this in my salons every day. The smiles of my satisfied clients reflect more than just momentary satisfaction—there can be many more benefits in the weeks to come, both psychologically and socially.

On the other hand, let's consider why someone's hair might be messy or poorly coiffed. Let's assume that the person is not "anti-establishment" and trying to make a statement with outrageous and unconventional looks. Someone who neglects his or her hair is missing an opportunity to look and feel even better. And if there are self-image issues that need attention, a more suitable hairstyle or a well-chosen new color may make a dramatic and wonderful difference.

As we journey together through the six weeks of *The Park Avenue Diet*, you will learn even more about how to take care of your hair—and how to create a variety of styles suitable for a variety of different locations, situations, and activities. Don't be afraid to experiment, and don't be afraid to change. You can learn a great deal of wonderful things about yourself in the process.

BASIC PRINCIPLES OF FABULOUS HAIR

The basic elements of a hairstyle are the length, color, texture and type. There are endless possibilities; even subtle changes to one element can change your whole look. In addition, it's important to learn how your environment affects your coiffeur and how to maintain healthy tresses.

1.

Know when your hairstyle has outgrown its ideal length.

Short hair cuts are easy to style and great in the summer to keep your hair off your neck. But you need to develop an inner barometer for determining when your hairstyle has outgrown its boundaries and your hair has reached an uncomfortable level.

Long hair can be more versatile. If you have straight hair, you can go for a cut that has more layers and angles to change the style without cutting it off. If you have curly hair, you can straighten it "pin straight," or leave a slight wave that will look bouncy and very pretty. Natural curls can also be lovely with the right setting gel to keep the curls in shape and lock in moisture to prevent frizz (avoid a "crunchy curl," which looks wet but actually dries hair further).

Long and medium-length hair can be gathered into a ponytail for a sporty look, or, for something more chic, pulled into a simple bun. The trick with medium-length hair is to know how to work with it. Practice wearing it up, down, wavy or straight. Have fun with it!

2.

Choose a hair color that matches your personality.

There is a strong psychological component to hairstyles, and different colors signal different emotions to everyone. Redheads, for instance, are unique, a minority of the people we see daily. A redhead therefore has a unique opportunity to stand out: if the style could speak it would be saying "look at me."

If you want brunette or black hair, be sure never to go more than three shades lighter or darker than your real color in order for the shade to look natural.

In contrast, it's wrong for someone to have overprocessed blond hair just to get attention. Good blond hair should have a casual look—the person will have no trouble getting attention the right way.

3.

Experiment with different textures and types.

You needn't drastically cut your hair in order to achieve a different look. Instead, you can try to alter the texture or type of your hair. There are four basic textures—*fine, medium, coarse,* or *wiry*—and four basic types—*straight, curly, wavy,* or *kinky*. In addition, your hair may be *normal, oily, dry, damaged,* or a *combination*. To a certain extent, the texture, type, and condition of your hair is determined by genetics, but hair products and your efforts can alter these conditions if you'd like. For example, all types of chemical process will alter texture. Coloring will give a rougher texture (beneficial to fine hair); chemical relaxer will make coarse/wiry hair smoother. You can change hair type with products that, for example, straighten curls or create them.

4.

Act your age.

Expert stylists take age into consideration when designing your "look." I'm sure that you don't want to look older than you actually are—you'd appear dowdy, which is hardly flattering. On the other hand, hairstyles that are right for younger people could make someone older seem insecure or like they're trying too hard. "Act your age," we are told from childhood, and it's true at every point in our lives. Wearing your hair like you are still in high school only works for a limited time after your graduation. Don't try to fool anyone about your age—instead, dazzle them with how good you look, no matter how old you are.

5.

Pay attention to your environment.

Your environment affects your hair, and we're talking here about nature, not your social world.

Exposure to sunlight, for instance, which gives a healthy glow to the skin, can be bad for your hair. If you've colored your hair, sunlight can actually lighten your hair and in effect change the colors. If you haven't colored your hair and you have dark hair, the sun will bring out natural highlights, which might soften your appearance and actually look great—or, give you a color you don't like. That's why, to protect your color from lightening due to sunlight exposure, use a product with SPF. Of course, you might also use a hair shield—or simply wear a hat.

Humidity—the amount of moisture in the air—can also affect your hair, causing it to frizz and act up. Control frizzy hair by using a hair polish or calming serum before blow-drying your hair. The effects of wintry weather, cold and dry, should be avoided by using a deep conditioner once a week.

During the summer, hair damage may result from swimming in chlorinated pools. This dries your hair as significantly as exposure to bitter cold—with an added negative influence. Bleached hair is porous, and when the chlorine gets into your hair and you sit in the sun, it oxidizes your hair, and you risk developing a green tint.

6.

Invest in the right hair accessories.

It's crucially important that you have the right hair accessories in your home and learn to use them effectively. Let's begin by focusing on the hair dryer, an indispensable item for every household. While it's true that air drying avoids the risk of the damages caused by heated tools, our busy schedules often dictate other choices. The advantage to blow drying your hair is that you are able to achieve a smoother, more styled, volumized look. Hold the blow dryer about three inches away from your hair to avoid excessive exposure.

Hair brushes are also essential items, but be sure to buy quality products. You need to use a hair brush because it removes dead hairs. A good boar bristle brush also massages the scalp, increasing blood flow, which is good for your hair shaft. A great time to comb your hair is when you're in the shower and you have conditioner in. This will help your comb slide through more easily, resulting in less breakage. Also important to have are hair clasps that don't pull or break your hair.

Curly hair requires specialized attention. We've moved away from the exclusive use of curling irons over the past several decades, adding in hot rollers. When you use a product which is heat activated, both will help you achieve the curls you want with the protection your hair needs.

Some people like to straighten curly hair, mostly for a change. When you have curly hair you might straighten it for a sleeker, more polished look. When straightening your hair, use a product that will help set the look, as well as something to protect your hair from heat damage. Straightening tools can get very hot and cause your hair to break. After applying the necessary products, take small sections and work from the middle of your hair's length to the end.

SELF-ASSESSMENT OF HAIR HEALTH AND STYLES

Answer True or False to each statement, and see below to determine how much you know about hair health and hairstyles.

1. Most people have either an entirely dry or oily scalp—as well as entirely straight or curly hair.
2. You should brush from the bottom of your hair to the roots.
3. The very opposite of your natural color could never be the best and most appealing look for a change.
4. Gray hair looks good on a woman with confidence.
5. Too much hairspray or products with alcohol can make your hair look dull and unhealthy.
6. You need to have a haircut every six to eight weeks, regardless of the

color, length, or texture of your hair.

7. A boar bristle brush is rarely needed for home use.
8. Massage your scalp once a week to promote the circulation in the scalp.
9. Volumizers are a must for people with thinning hair.
10. Steam rooms are dangerous for one's hair.

The following statements are true: 2, 4, 5, 6, and 9.

The following statements are false: 1, 3, 7, 8, and 10.

If you answered more than five questions correctly, congratulations! Your hair already probably looks great, but we're going to take it up another level. If you answered fewer than five questions correctly, please start experimenting with various hair products; visit a good stylist to begin.

PARK AVENUE GROOMING
WITH LAURA GELLER

ABOUT LAURA GELLER

Laura Geller is one of the most highly respected and successful experts in makeup and beauty throughout the United States. The key to her success seems to lie somewhere in between her beauty expertise and her affable, approachable, and "best friend in the biz" personality. Not happy just being one of the industry's most recognized and talented makeup artists, Laura has made a career out of infusing glamour into every girl's day with innovative, functional products that are easy to use and easier to fall in love with.

From an early age, Laura knew her future would be in makeup. "I used to ask if I could work at the makeup counters for free just so I could be near the products," she explains. Her path to becoming one of the industry's top makeup artists swiftly followed as she went from beauty school to Broadway where she made up theater's rising stars. Soon after, Geller's handiwork was gracing the small screen, including on-air talent at CBS, NBC, AMC, and HBO.

In 1993, success struck again as Laura opened Laura Geller Makeup Studios on New York City's posh Upper East Side. The studio's purpose was simple: teach women the how-to of cosmetics and hands-on technique to master it. Laura sought to simplify makeup application. "I saw a void in the makeup industry. Women didn't know how to apply makeup, so I wanted to communicate my knowledge and experience," she says. Today, the studio is a showcase for Laura's eponymous line of cosmetics and is also where those in the know flock for five-star makeup application, brow shaping, and more. You can find Laura's products for sale on QVC and in Sephora stores nationwide.

WHY GROOMING AND MAKEUP ARE IMPORTANT TO
THE PARK AVENUE DIET

When you enter a room, what do you think people should notice first? Your clothing, your hairstyle, your self-confidence, your interpersonal skills, your physique, your weight, or your makeup? The answer should be obvious: just like Frank Sinatra sang, "All or nothing at all."

People view us as a totality of the components of our image, and no single aspect should be flawed. This is particularly true when we discuss makeup. It should never be obvious yet it must reflect and enhance our positive inner feelings.

I began my career in the theater, where makeup is used for dramatic purposes to define certain character traits. In the real world, makeup is a good way to bolster self-confidence—it helps us play the part of our smarter and sexier self. And improved self-confidence is a great way to make us more careful in how we treat our bodies.

BECOME YOUR OWN MAKEUP ARTIST

Would you like to learn how to apply makeup like a celebrity? Here's how: find a reputable cosmetic department within your local department store, or a private makeup studio that offers expert advice. Invest the time and money if needed so you can learn and get advice from a reputable cosmetic counter. Find out who does makeup lessons or look closely at a magazine. Keep the photo close by and try similar colors. Test it out first. Don't be in a hurry. You can become your own makeup artist with enough time and care.

You can start with these basics. Let's focus first on your eyes. They are the windows to your soul. Not surprisingly, they are what most people look at first, perhaps a way of entering your philosophical and psychological world.

Eyeshadow is one of the primary tools in cosmetics. It is used to create shape, angularity, and sculpting; it actually can make eyes look larger and more defined. Think of the spectacular effect that Elizabeth Taylor created as Cleopatra. For everyday purposes, however, pick a wearable shade that is neither bright nor loud. If your makeup tends to fade, consider using a fade-resistant shadow, or buy primers you can put on your eyelids before you apply eyeshadow.

Now take a closer look at your eyebrows. They are the framework of your eyes. Proper shaping of your eyebrows speaks to how well-groomed you are. If you can, I urge you to go for a professional brow shaping on a regular basis to maintain that perfect shape.

Use eyebrow pencil carefully to create the proper framework and shape of your eyebrows. On your eyelid, eyeliner should be applied along the base of your lashline (top and bottom lashes) to enhance the shape of your eyes. Mascara makes eyelashes look fuller and more youthful. But don't get carried away; people should not look at your lashes because you have on too much mascara. Try to avoid waterproof mascara, which will dry out your lashes; instead, use water-resistant mascara.

Lipstick is a mood enhancer, "whatever moves you." Put on a bold color if you're feeling funky; it might change your mood for the better.

Foundations come in all textures and delivery systems today. You may even find several that work well for your complexion. Remember, it may be a matter of trial and error before you find the right product. The foundation you choose should never look cakey.

Blush is intended to add color to your skintone and should be applied to make your cheekbones look more sculpted. Generally, blush is available in shades of pink, mauve, warm coral, and bronzes. Your skin is not just one tone, so you may want a mixture of more than one color to use for blush.

A NOTE ABOUT MAKEUP BRUSHES

Makeup brushes and applicators are as important as the actual makeup. The proper tools help makeup look more polished and finished. People often ask me "Which are the most important makeup tools?" Here's my list:

1. Eyeshadow brushes: if an eyeshadow brush has the right shape and hairs, you will get better ease of use.
2. Natural, non-latex sponges to blend out foundations or concealers.

3. Blush brushes to define cheekbones to give the face a sculpted look.

By the way, be sure to clean makeup brushes often, especially complexion brushes that you are regularly putting on your face like blush or powder brushes (and don't forget your eyeliner brushes as well). Wipe the brushes and use antibacterial liquid once a week.

BASIC PRINCIPLES OF GROOMING

1.

Your skin is your canvas.

Just like an artist, you must create something that draws attention yet is subtle at the same time. But first, your skin needs to be smooth and blank. You must make sure to have the best possible "clean slate." It is the preparation for the rest to come. You don't want to use makeup to cover up but to enhance. Nevertheless, you need to get your skin in perfect order first.

2.

Approach makeup as an accessory to your wardrobe.

Just as your clothing choices must reflect your hair color, age, physique, and self-concept, your makeup choices also must reflect multiple aspects of facial features, inner feelings, and your social environment.

3.

The skin is a bodily organ.

The cells of your skin are continuously regenerated and sloughed off. Moreover, there are many layers of skin, each with its own texture and function.

Your head is not a sphere. Take a careful look and you will see that the left and right sides of your face are slightly different. In other words, learning about makeup includes learning about symmetry.

4.

Your skin should look as if you are not wearing makeup.

This may seem like an unusual statement coming from a makeup expert like me. However, I never want to view someone solely based on the makeup she is wearing. Instead, I want to see the shape of her eyes, cheekbones, and lips enhanced by makeup.

5.

Concealing facial flaws restores our sense of integrity.

Using the proper products and application techniques, we can get rid of redness around the nose, dark circles around the eyes, and unsightly blemishes. Then we can approach the world. Concealers come in all shapes, sizes, and textures depending on how much coverage you need: the thicker the concealer, the more coverage you will get.

Piling on makeup can actually make blemishes look worse. Less is more when it comes to coverage. Blemishes are raised imperfections. We can cover discolorations, not raised areas. Because a blemish is raised, the makeup does not blend easily and you call more attention to the lesion. You can cover redness but you can not conceal a raised imperfection.

6.

Women need a personalized approach to makeup.

Every woman has her own style, which applies to clothing, hair, and self-image as well. Our look can be different for different social events, though. I also urge women to "break out of the box" for fun, too, and make a change to their "look." We never have to restrict ourselves to just one style.

7.

Learn from the women around you.

Let's face it: women always look at other women. And there's no harm in asking someone, "What are you wearing?" That's actually a great compliment. This is a way for women to help each other build self-confidence and move light-years ahead in happiness and achievement.

8.

Makeup is not for covering up: it's for enhancement.

A fortunate few people look good without makeup. They still need to be generally healthy and take care of their skin. But for most women, makeup is a technique of *chiaroscuro*, the skillful use of shading that balances out facial features. As the name implies, it is an art.

9.

Stress frequently affects the skin first.

Facial blemishes are sometimes the direct result of our environment and the stress we may endure. Learning how to cope with stress can be the best first step in dealing with some cosmetic issues. If personal stress is mirrored in your appearance, please deal with both the dermatological and psychological aspects at the same time.

10.

Be prepared to re-evaluate your makeup choices frequently and don't be afraid to experiment.

Let experts show you new looks and products that may take your appearance and spirits where they have never gone before.

SELF-ASSESSMENT OF GROOMING HABITS

Answer True or False to each statement, and see below to determine how much you know about grooming and makeup.

1. Most people have either an entirely dry or entirely oily skin type.
2. Exfoliation, promoting the loss of the outer layers of epidermis, is a way of deep cleaning and rejuvenating the skin.
3. Lipstick color should be changed to reflect or improve your mood.
4. Sculpting or contouring is a fine art that can define facial features.
5. You can test foundation or concealer color on your hands.
6. The skin on your face is the least susceptible to the aging process.
7. If you touch your face and makeup transfers to your hand or tissue, you need more makeup.
8. Acne can be effectively treated with new prescription medications, so consult a dermatologist.
9. Few male celebrities know how to use makeup, such as bronzers, effectively.
10. There are different makeup styles for each season.

The following statements are true: 2, 3, 4, 8, and 10
The following statements are false: 1, 5, 6, 7, and 9.
If you answered more than five questions correctly, congratulations! Your makeup already probably looks great, but we're going to take it up another level. If you answered fewer than five questions correctly, please start experimenting with basic makeup lesson in this chapter.

PARK AVENUE INTERPERSONAL SKILLS WITH TINSLEY MORTIMER

ABOUT TINSLEY MORTIMER

Tinsley Mortimer's rise to the top of New York society was inevitable due to her winning combination of charitable contributions, elegant beauty, and entrepreneurial savvy. Born in Richmond, Virginia, she received a baccalaureate degree in art history at Columbia University, has excelled at tennis, and worked in major fashion and public relations organizations. A true Park Avenue resident, she is the best guide you could have for *The Park Avenue Diet*.

WHY INTERPERSONAL SKILLS ARE IMPORTANT TO *THE PARK AVENUE DIET*

How you feel about yourself is reflected in how you interact with other people. If you have a negative approach to life's problems and have neglected your appearance, it will be difficult to convince people that you are someone worth knowing.

Maybe you are not the tallest or the prettiest person, but this is your one chance on Earth to enjoy the beauty of life. And one of life's greatest joys is the blessing of companionship, the bonds between you and others, whether friends, family, or new acquaintances. Close, honest relationships will in turn make you a happier person and will also make you want to focus even more carefully on your appearance and behavior. Besides, it's fun to have wonderful friends.

Interpersonal skills all depend on a single principle of human behavior: it's easier to be nice. Ever notice that when you are smiling, you stop focusing inwardly and brooding on problems? We all will have our share of difficult problems, but no one wants to add yours to his or her own. A smile is a message of warmth and empathy, so let your positive feelings be the first type of greeting you offer others.

Some people reduce interpersonal skills to a single word, politeness, but this is a limited definition of a very important component of your image. Your outward behavior cannot be different from your innermost feelings; otherwise, social skills are merely a façade, an acting performance. Good interpersonal skills cannot be part of a hidden agenda; be nice for the sake of being nice.

People always gravitate to individuals who are joyous, uplifting, and sunny. Your innermost feelings can easily be "read" on the outside, as mirrored by your facial expressions, hand gestures, and body language. The more you love yourself—and prove this by taking care of yourself—the more others will want to be your friends. And give everyone a chance. You will never know how many amazing people surround you unless you truly give everyone a chance to be your friend—a chance that you may actually like them and their companionship. Our world seems smaller than ever, and you will have the opportunity to meet people from many different backgrounds. Do not judge people beforehand, quickly, or superficially; try to like them and get to know them as individuals, not stereotypyes or two-dimensional characters.

You should have no ulterior motives for treating people with kindness, humility, and respect. Being uplifting, optimistic, and inspiring may develop as an inner philosophy, but when applied to your social behavior, it serves as a source of strength, comfort, and attraction to those around you. Good energy draws people closer; negative energy drives people away.

LISTENING, A VERY IMPORTANT INTERPERSONAL SKILL

Interpersonal skills are not necessarily overt actions, like warmly shaking someone's hand or answering a phone call with a smile (you'll sound happier). One of the most important, for example, is being a good listener. This is as important as being a good speaker, and each person should be 50% of every conversation. Your friends need to know that you have the patience, empathy, and interest to hear their opinions and to be a sounding board for their problems.

Being a good listener also includes keeping others' comments in confidence. It is important that your friends know that they can count on you in difficult times and that they may speak honestly and openly with no fear that their words will be repeated. If asked for your opinions, be truthful and sensitive. Keep your remarks brief and respectful, letting people know that they need to trust their own judgment. A good listener is a good adviser and a good friend.

Lose yourself in someone's world when he or she is speaking to you; then you will be able to listen attentively and understand the problems at hand, without interrupting to share a similar story. Let the other person finish what he or she is saying. You may give your opinion, but do not insist that your solution is the only way. Do not burden the other individual with a list of your own personal problems; this behavior is very insensitive and offers no useful solutions or insights, just self-centeredness.

Make sure that your philosophy of life and the way you treat others are in harmony. Also be sure that people have a positive experience from being with you. Good behavior must emanate from good feelings, about others and about yourself. The Golden Rule ("Do unto others as you would have others do unto you.") has inspired generations since the words were first written, and in the complex, fast-moving world of today, this truism is perhaps more powerful than ever. Living with a conscience, with morals and integrity, is as important as the routine tasks you do every day. Making other people happy and brightening their lives are not arcane ideals that are obsolete in a highly technological world. The more you reflect the beauty and joy of life, the more rewards you can receive—but expect nothing in return. Be sincere, be inclusive, be respectful, and be positive.

BASIC PRINCIPLES OF INTERPERSONAL SKILLS

1. Everyone needs interpersonal skills, regardless of where they come from.
2. You won't have staying power without interpersonal skills. You may get somewhere on your own, but you need to stay there, and getting along with others is essential to success.
3. The way people respond to you will make your life better and make you a stronger person. This will be reflected in your personal appearance as well.
4. Interpersonal skills develop as you get older. The goal—people want to be your friend.
5. Treat others as you would like to be treated. Your social skills reflect your inner beliefs and your feelings about yourself.
6. People will pay more attention to you when you make them feel good about themselves, but don't use flattery for your own enrichment. Do it because you want to be nice, and you want people to enjoy being with you.
7. Show respect to everyone. Even a person in the lowest imaginable job is a human being with feelings.
8. Don't live by worrying "What do they think of me?" People are usually thinking about themselves.
9. Don't put on a façade when you interact with other people. Everyone wants to know "the real you," so be optimistic, pleasant, and honest.
10. Attention to body language is as important an interpersonal skill as proper choice of words and courtesy. Your eyes and hands reflect your thoughts, so be friendly and sincere at all times.

SOUTHERN HOSPITALITY TIPS

Growing up in Virginia included a great deal of attention to social skills that are an intrinsic part of the culture. "Hospitality" is no different from the way individuals should treat each other anywhere, but we were taught this on a personal and a community level. Inclusiveness, whether it means inviting someone to your home or maintaining good eye contact in a conversation, is a way of making others feel happy. And caring about others—even putting their feelings before yours—is what life is all about.

What we were taught as considerate behavior is indeed a way of showing respect, deference, and empathy. Here are some examples that are commonplace courtesies in Virginia. In the appropriate setting, some may enhance your other interpersonal skills.

1.   You should always stand when an older person comes to your table or enters the room, whether you are a man or a woman.

2.   Southerners occasionally gently touch people while in conversation with their friends. Just a little touch on the forearm says "I like you and I am really listening to you." Combined with a warm smile and good conversational skills, it's a small gesture that reflects sincere inner feelings.

3.   When introducing people to each other, first introduce the younger person to the older person. For example, "Mrs. Winslow, I would like you to meet my friend Fabiola. Fabiola, this is mother's dear friend Mrs. Winslow." And when someone approaches you and you are in a group of people, make sure that the people know the person approaching. Otherwise, introduce the newcomer to your group: "Fabiola, these are my friends Lauren and Amanda. Lauren and Amanda, this is my friend Fabiola." or this way: "Everyone, you all know Fabiola Baracasa, don't you?" Then let each member of the group introduce herself or himself.

4.   If you have been the guest in someone's home, have received a present, or have simply been treated specially, always send a thank-you note on lovely stationery. It doesn't matter how large the present is or how significant the favor seems. Appreciation can be a present too, so take extra time to show your warm feelings. This holds true even for close members of your family, especially your grandparents. Put down that Blackberry—e-mails are inadequate.

SELF-ASSESSMENT OF INTERPERSONAL SKILLS

Before you begin *The Park Avenue Diet*, take a few minutes to assess your knowledge of interpersonal skills. Decide whether the following statements are true or false:

1. Someone's "personal space" or "comfort zone" refers only to the physical distance between that individual and other people.
2. A conversation should never be monopolized by one person.
3. You'll learn more about yourself and your capabilities if you confine your friendships to people exactly like you.
4. Arguments are an ineffective and upsetting way of dealing with relationship issues.
5. Nonverbal communication (such as gestures, tone of voice, facial expressions and posture) is far less important than the words you use while conversing with other people.
6. It is not necessary to be tactful around your friends; they need to accept you the way you are.
7. A sincere "thank you" is one of the most important phrases in the English language for developing and maintaining friendships.
8. It is old-fashioned and outdated to say "after you," and to open the door for people when you enter a building.
9. Being a good listener requires sincere interest in the feelings and thoughts of others, not merely momentary attention.
10. Developing closer relationships can also improve your own self-confidence and attention to personal appearance.

The following statements are true: 2, 4, 7, 9, and 10.

The following statements are false: 1, 3, 5, 6, and 8.

If you answered more than five questions correctly, congratulations! You probably have good friends and an active social life, but we'll help you feel more comfortable in any social situation. If you answered fewer than five questions correctly, please review this chapter carefully and keep the basic principles in mind as you talk with new and old friends.

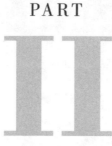

PART

II

THE SIX-WEEK
PARK AVENUE DIET

*N*ow that you've learned the basic principles of the seven areas of image reinvention, it's time to start putting them into action. In this part, we've given you a day-by-day plan to help you incorporate healthy new habits, fashionable new styles, and positive new ways of thinking into your everyday life.

Because diet and exercise are crucial parts of any weight-loss plan, you'll see that we've given you a suggested menu and workout for every day. Although you can certainly get results if you work out only three times a week, as Bernadette indicated, initially it will help to do a little bit every day in order to get into the fitness habit. To get you started, this plan will begin with one exercise a day until you build up to a full interval training circuit. If you already exercise regularly, good for you! Keep it up, add Bernadette's exercises to your routine, and you'll see results even faster.

The suggested menus from Chef Marie are designed to give you balanced nutrition, a variety of flavors, and, most importantly, pleasure in your meals. Each day's menus add up to approximately 1200 to 1500 calories, but I don't want you to focus only on counting calories or portions. Keep in mind that the suggested menus are just suggestions, so feel free to vary them to suit your tastes.

Remember that you don't need to cook everything on this suggested list. Leftovers can be used as substitutes throughout the week, or you can use the quickest snack and meal suggestions if you are pressed for time. If you are allergic to a particular item or have a special favorite from the recipe list, make an appropriate substitution—as long as you stick to *The Park Avenue Diet*.

As for beverages, mineral water is your best bet, not milk, juice, soda, or "vitamin" water. Recent controversial studies suggest that diet sodas might actually promote obesity rather than "cure" it; in any case, they are chemical concoctions devoid of nutritional benefit. Need a cup of caffeinated coffee or tea in the morning? Go ahead, but add only skim milk if necessary, never sugar or artificial sweeteners.

Finally, each day you will get additional advice on improving your appearance—with a fashion, hair, or grooming tip—and guidance on changing your behavior by boosting your self-confidence or enhancing your interpersonal skills.

The plan has three phases. Phase 1, Inviting Success, which takes two weeks, is a self-discovery stage; you'll learn how to apply each of the seven components to your personal situation and goals. In Phase 2, Preparing for Greatness, which is just a week, you'll be practicing your newfound skills. And finally, in Phase 3, Making the A-List, you'll unveil the new you. We suggest that you begin the plan on a Saturday so that you'll have more time in the first couple of days of each phase to devote to the plan, but you can start whenever works best for you.

Now let's get started!

MENU

Meal	Recipe	Yield	Calories	P. No.
Breakfast	Country Frittata	(1 serving)	230	153
Lunch	Chicken Salad with Fruit	(1 serving)	376	194
Snack	Olive Paste and Tomato Bruschetta or 1/2 pink/red grapefruit	(2 servings)	136 (53 for 1/2 grapefruit)	197
Dinner	Tuna Provencal	(1 serving)	328	155
Dessert	Winter Fruit Salad	(1 serving)	135	201
Total			1205	

EXERCISE

The Squat: We'll start off with this compound exercise, one that works many muscle groups at the same time. You'll be strengthening your quadriceps, hamstrings, glutes, and calves—and virtually all muscles from the waist down. Please take the time to learn this important exercise well—it's the mack daddy of them all!

1. Stand up straight like a soldier, with your head and shoulders back and down and chest raised. Your feet are shoulder-width or slightly farther apart, toes pointed slightly out.
2. Tuck your abs in (tuck your belly button into your lower back), inhale and lower down as if you are sitting onto a chair behind you (not straight down). Your arms can extend straight out in front at shoulder height, or you may hold light weights at your sides. Keep your knees in line with your feet (not bowed in or out) and check to make sure the knees don't extend past your toes. Your head looks forward, not up or down, as you lower your thighs parallel to the floor, or as close to that as possible. Heels stay down.
3. When you've reached parallel, hold for a moment, then exhale and come back up to standing position, tilting your pelvis forward and up as you ascend. Keep the knees unlocked.

Every rep should be challenging, but concentrate on getting the form correct today. If you feel unsteady, you can actually touch your bottom to a couch. This will serve as a marker to show you how deep to squat while helping you feel balanced and secure.

Aim to do 12 squats slowly and carefully, and check your form in a mirror. Make sure that your thighs are parallel to the floor, so you look like you're sitting down onto a bench, and your abs are tucked in. Your goal today is three sets of 12 squats (or as many as possible until fatigued) with regular breathing, proper alignment, and, of course, a smile. Keep your eyes straight ahead.

Exercise	Reps	Sets
Squats	12— or as many as possible until fatigued	3

FASHION TIP

Organize: As you begin to slim down, you will need to invest in new clothing that matches the new you. Start preparing now: throw out tattered items and donate outdated clothing. Replace wire hangers with quality wood hangers that will keep your clothes looking newer longer.

SELF-CONFIDENCE SKILLS

Write down the exact words that go through your mind when you crave a certain type of food or when you overeat. For example:

"A cookie right now would help me take my mind off my depression."
"Just one handful of potato chips won't add very much weight to my body."
"If I go on a splurge tonight, I can fast all day tomorrow."
"I deserve that extra dessert for all the hard work I did today."

Now, find a substitute phrase that you can use to counter that thought and feeling:

"It is better for me to find the source of my depression and work it through, rather than to distract myself with junk food."
"I know that I won't be able to stop with one handful, so it is better not to start at all."
"I know from my experience that I will forget about fasting tomorrow."
"I deserve to keep weight off. That is a better reward than binge eating."

Throughout your journey of self-discovery and reinvention, you will be getting in touch with your incorrect, unreasoned, and often self-destructive personal myths, rewriting them into positive statements that will inspire you to attain self-fulfillment and better health.

Phase 1 | INVITING SUCCESS

MENU

Meal	Recipe	Yield	Calories	P. No.
Breakfast	Sweet Bell Pepper and Spinach Omelet	(1 serving)	224	152
Lunch	Pasta with Vegetables and Sundried Tomatoes	(1 serving)	347	181
Snack	Dip 10 baby carrots in 1 tablespoon tapenade		110	TK
Dinner	Chicken with Mushrooms	(1 serving)	402	165
	Brown Rice Pilaf	(1 serving)		180
Dessert	Have 2 sliced fresh peaches topped with 1 tablespoon each chopped walnuts and slivered almonds		178	
Total			1261	

EXERCISE

The Push-Up: Today we'll focus on this classic and fantastic component of your workout, one that also requires perfect form to achieve maximal results. You'll be strengthening your chest, shoulders, and arms, particularly the triceps. Beginners: try this with your knees on the ground or standing up, pressing against a wall as if it were the floor.

1. Lie with your hands at shoulder level, palms flat on the floor slightly more than shoulder width apart. Your feet are parallel to each other and close together. Look forward (not down at floor) and keep your body straight, toes tucked under your feet. If you are on your knees, keep a straight line from shoulders to knees, and let the tops of your feet rest on the floor behind you.
2. Exhale, straighten your arms, and push up off the floor. Palms stay put, tummy is tucked, and body is straight. No arches or bends in the back, please. Pause for a moment at the top.
3. Inhale, and lower your body back to 2 inches from the floor (or wall)—pause and repeat.

Voila! You've learned another terrific powerhouse exercise that you can do virtually anywhere! Do as many reps as you can in each set—for beginners that may only be 3 to 6 at first—so be it. You'll quickly add on as you keep doing these. And I'd rather see you do 6 proper-form pushups than do 20 mis-performed movements, because with proper form you will see results much faster.

Exercise	Reps	Sets
Push-Ups	As many as possible until fatigued	3

HAIR TIP

How often should you shampoo or condition your hair, and what should you use? It really depends on what kind of hair you have. If you have oily hair you should be washing your hair once a day to remove the oils that weigh your hair down. If you have dry hair you should wash your hair every other day and use a deep conditioning treatment or a product like a daily hair masque.

But if you have very dry hair, use a deep conditioner periodically, applying a product rich in vitamins to the ends of your hair. Flat hair that needs fuller body and volume? Use a volumizing shampoo and conditioner. Also, apply a volumizing spray to the root of your hair and blow-dry. You should always start blow-drying at the root in order for the hair to be completely dry all around. The direction you blow-dry is the direction your hair will take on—for example, blowing hair upward will give more volume at crown/roots. And if you pull downward, you will get a smoother, straighter look.

INTERPERSONAL SKILLS

People who are the "center of attention" are, by definition, surrounded by admirers throughout the day, whether at school, at the mall, or at a party. Magnetic and attractive individuals have therefore mastered the skills of both verbal and nonverbal "mass communication"; they know how to be the focus of attention in a group, even as they talk with only one person.

How is it possible to speak with one person and simultaneously rivet the attention of others? Simply put, be inclusive, and be sure to give everyone around you a little "face time."

Today, when you have an opportunity to share a conversation with several friends or co-workers, make a conscious effort to acknowledge and look at everyone in the group. When speaking to one person, you should establish eye contact, even if briefly, with the others. No one likes to feel left out, so make sure that each listener receives a smile and momentary attention.

Hollywood stars on the "red carpet" wave and smile to fans in every direction. It illustrates the magnitude of their popularity. If you want to be someone that everyone wants to know better, practice this skill today. Speak to one group member with your voice and to the others with your eyes and smile.

Phase 1 | INVITING SUCCESS

INVITING SUCCESS

Phase 1

MENU

Meal	Recipe	Yield	Calories	P. No.
Breakfast	Homemade Granola with Pumpkin Yogurt	(1 serving)	313	148
Lunch	Beet Salad	(1 serving)	278	190
Snack	Have 1 tablespoon dried cranberries or blueberries with 2 tablespoons chopped walnuts		123	
Dinner	Broiled Tuna with Tarragon Sauce	(1 serving)	264 134	157
	Brown Rice Pilaf	(1 serving)		180
Dessert	Chocolate Square with Raspberry Coulis, or one plum	(1 serving)	138 (30 calories for plum)	203
Total			1250	

EXERCISE

Bent-Over Back Row: Today we'll learn another great compound exercise that works your middle back and biceps, while helping to develop terrific posture. We "pushed" with the push-up and now will "pull" with this rowing movement to balance and naturally stretch the muscles in opposition. You'll need light weights, starting with two pound to five pound handweights and adding more weight when 12 reps done with proper form becomes easy.

1. Stand up straight with your chest out proudly, shoulders back and down. Feet are slightly more than shoulder-width apart.
2. Bend forward at your waist (about a 60-degree angle) so that your chest is over your feet and knees are slightly bent. Your tummy is tucked in and your head is looking forward—not down. Arms are fully extended to knees or shins, and your hands hold the weights so your thumbs point in toward one another.
3. Exhale, squeeze your back muscles, and then slowly lift or "row" the weights up to the outer rib-cage area. Squeeze your shoulder blades together as you go. Keep your head up and looking forward, tummy tucked in, and shoulders back throughout exercise to help keep your back stable and firm.
4. Pause, inhale and lower the weights back down slowly to starting position. Repeat. Remember to keep the head up and shoulders back the whole way through. Engage the back muscles first—then the arms—to get the most "bang for buck." Think: "the back is the boss and the arms are the assistants" for this movement. Good work!.

If you find this difficult, try it first without the weights. Do this exercise 12 times or as many reps as possible until fatigued.

Exercise	Reps	Sets
Back Row	12 or as many as possible until fatigued	1

GROOMING TIP

Determine your skin type. If you have dry, dehydrated skin, your skin will feel tight, like it needs moisture. Sometimes it will lack luster or vitality and may flake. Usually mature and/or fair skin (skin that burns easily) is dry. If your skin has large pores, is shiny or subject to breakouts, your skin is oily. If you have olive skin, it's probably normal or oily. Breakouts on olive or darker complexions tend to give the skin a shiny look. Almost everyone has combination skin. One area (usually the T-zone—nose, forehead, chin) may be oily, and the rest of the skin may be dry. Pores in the T-zone may have blackheads, and more breakouts will occur there.

For dry skin, exfoliation should be very limited. Only use serums around the eyes, not heavier creams.

For oily skin, exfoliate before putting on makeup. Use liquid cleansers and oil-free lotion for moisturizing, rather than heavy creams.

SELF-CONFIDENCE SKILLS

It is not enough to identify unhealthy personal myths and come up with statements that support a healthy lifestyle. In addition, you need to examine the underlying feelings that accompany the words. So take each of the statements from yesterday and ask yourself, "How do I feel when those words go through my mind?"

For example, many people tell themselves, "If I go on a splurge tonight I can fast all day tomorrow." They feel good about this resolution because it gives them permission to go on an eating binge. But the next day, they usually "forget" about fasting because they are too busy or are tempted by new food choices.

You might discover that you feel like rebelling whenever you make a resolution. Perhaps you rebelled against suggestions and advice when you were a child. That rebellion served a purpose, making you into an individual who did not blindly follow commands issued by parents, siblings, or peers. But it makes no sense for you to rebel against your own decisions.

Whenever you feel like rebelling, just direct that feeling toward the people who want you to overeat, toward the advertisements that urge you to buy high-calorie food, and the restaurants that serve you super-sized meals. In other words, don't fight your feelings, simply redirect them in ways that will help you drop the pounds and keep them from returning.

Phase 1 | INVITING SUCCESS

MENU

Meal	Recipe	Yield	Calories	P. No.
Breakfast	All-Bran with Apples and Cinnamon	(1 serving)	252	146
Lunch	Pasta with Vegetables and Sundried Tomatoes	(1 serving)	347	181
Snack	Have 2 tablespoons sunflower seeds and 1 tablespoon dried blueberries		127	
Dinner	Chicken au Citron	(1 serving)	245	167
	Zucchini and Bell Peppers with Pine Nuts	(1 serving)	117	176
Dessert	Thin Apple Tart	(1 serving)	160	205
Total			1248	

EXERCISE

The Lunge: These can be thought of as one-legged squats, superb exercises for your legs, glutes, and core muscles. First, get the form down perfectly:

1. Put your front foot flat on the floor and your back foot 2 feet back, resting on the toe, heel off the floor.
2. Lower the rear knee toward the floor, inhaling as you do so, and pause.
3. Press up with front leg, exhaling as you do so and rising in a straight line. Look carefully—the front knee must be directly over the front ankle at all times.

If you need to hold on to a table or desk for balance, go right ahead. Alternatively, you may prefer to hold your hands at your sides or to flex your elbows as a counterbalance. Form is extremely important, so check yourself out in a mirror occasionally.

Let's start with 12 times for the left leg, then 12 lunges for the right leg. Our goal for today: three sets of 12 lunges for each leg—slowly, carefully, with perfect form. Now go to it—I'm watching you!

Exercise	Reps	Sets
Lunge	12 left leg / 12 right leg	3

FASHION TIP

Make an appointment to look at yourself in the mirror once, and only once, per day. A daily date with the mirror will allow you to constructively assess your appearance and style. Be sure to look at yourself from all angles before walking away feeling relaxed and confident.

INTERPERSONAL SKILLS

Conversation is not just a way to communicate with people; it's also a way to attract and befriend them. If you want to meet that special someone, your verbal skills will be extremely useful right at the start.

Always make sure the person you're talking with feels comfortable at all times. Be aware of his or her background and experiences and choose your topics accordingly. And remember: conversations are not all about you, so be a good listener as well. Avoid focusing on yourself, appearing extremely opinionated, or being overly revealing

Think of a conversation like a tennis match; the ball can only be on one side of the court at a time. Simply put: "You talk, they talk, you talk, they talk." When someone else is speaking, be attentive; maintain eye contact, smile, and wait until he or she has completed a sentence or thought before you take your turn.

Practice "you talk, they talk" today with a family member, a bus driver, or a teacher. Remember not to interrupt, and leave some "air space" between their sentence and yours. Be patient when speaking to people and show that you are sincerely interested in them.

Master this skill well, and be prepared for the very pleasant consequences.

Phase 1 | INVITING SUCCESS

MENU

Meal	Recipe	Yield	Calories	P. No.
Breakfast	Buckwheat Crêpes with Salmon	(1 serving)	181	150
Lunch	Salade Niçoise au Citron	(1 serving)	489	195
Snack	Dip 7 cherry tomatoes in 1 tablespoon olive tapenade		97	
Dinner	Salmon à l'Orange	(1 serving)	368	159
Dessert	Winter Fruit Salad	(1 serving)	135	201
Total			1270	

EXERCISE

The **Shoulder Press:** The shoulder press is terrific for your upper body. You'll need light weights (start with 2- to 5- pound hand weights).

1. Stand with one foot in front of another, 2 to 3 feet apart, then slightly bend the front knee and the back knee.
2. Lift the weights to shoulder level (the starting point) and then press straight up, exhaling as you do so, for a count of 2.
3. Inhale as you lower the weights back to shoulder level on a count of 4.

Your elbows are slightly bent at the top, not locked, and your legs stay in the bent knee position throughout the movement. Ideally, you should do 3 sets of 12 reps today.

Exercise	Reps	Sets
Shoulder Press	Aim for 12 or as many as possible until fatigued.	3

INVITING SUCCESS

Phase 1

HAIR TIP

Your hair can never be described with a single word. Your hair may be dry or oily, straight or curly, normal or damaged, or any combination of these.

How can you figure out if your hair is oily, dry, or healthy? The best way is to touch/feel your hair; if it's giving off oil in your hand, it's oily; if it's dry you'll know by frizzies all over, a dry, dehydrated feel, and dull look. "Healthy" hair will have an even; light coat of shine all over and feel strong, with minimal split ends to the naked eye. Combination hair will be straight, wavy, or curly in different areas. The best way to work with this type of hair is to figure out which type you want and alter it appropriately.

Once you properly decipher which type of hair you have and the product you need to manage it, be aware that you might need multiple products to tame several different problems.

If your hair is curly and frizzy you might want to use a smoothing shampoo and conditioner and hair polish; if your hair is dry and damaged you would want to use a nurturing shampoo and conditioner and strengthener.

Once you have determined the condition of your hair you will be able to properly treat it.

SELF-CONFIDENCE SKILLS

People who help to reinforce your new body image are often referred to as a "support group." Those who directly or indirectly undercut your new body image may be more comfortable with you the way you were. These people are also called "co-dependents." Like relatives or friends who keep supplying an addict with cigarettes, alcohol, or illegal drugs, food co-dependents keep bringing you high-calorie foods and express disappointment when you don't eat the cakes, cookies, muffins, and pastries that they have made or bought "just for you."

So cling to members of the support group who reinforce healthy eating habits. Keep a respectful distance from co-dependents whose personal myths favor carelessness rather than fitness, vitality, and well-being.

Phase 1 | INVITING SUCCESS

MENU

Meal	Recipe	Yield	Calories	P. No.
Breakfast	Orange Wheat Muffin	(1 serving)	202	151
Lunch	Spinach and Onion Soup	(2 servings)	394	185
Snack	Mix 6 ounces low-fat plain yogurt with 2 teaspoons dried blueberries or raisins		125	
Dinner	Chicken Cacciatora	(1 serving)	489	168
Dessert	Have 2 sliced fresh peaches topped with 1 tablespoon each chopped walnuts and slivered almonds		178	
Total			1388	

EXERCISE

The One-Arm Row: These are a slight variation on the back rows we learned on Day 3. You'll need light weights for one hand at a time.

1. Stand with your legs farther than hip-width apart with the knees slightly bent, holding a weight in one hand. Now, lean forward with a flat back, following the same form as in our previous back row exercise.
2. Lift the arm holding the weight, contracting your back/shoulder blade, not your elbow. Exhale as you lift to the outer rib cage area. Your free hand may rest on the knee in front of it.
3. Slowly lower your arm until completely extended, inhaling as you lower the weight.

Your goal: lift each arm in succession for 10–12 reps aiming for 3 sets.

Exercise	Reps	Sets
One-Arm row	12 left / 12 Right or until fatigued	3

GROOMING TIP

Be sure you are using the right skin cleanser for your skin type. For dry skin, use a gentle cleanser that has hydrating properties. Exfoliate twice a week with a gentle product, featuring papaya or enzymes, for example. You can also use a combination exfoliator/cleanser.

Those with oily skin can exfoliate more often, even every day, as long as they don't use a product that is too harsh. Be sure to use oil-free cleansers.

Combination skin requires a cleanser designed to address both conditions.

No matter what type of skin you have, the first step is always exfoliation. Exfoliation gets rid of dead skin cells. A note: apricot-based exfoliants are very harsh and are recommended only for very oily skin.

INTERPERSONAL SKILLS

"Too close for comfort" can describe your situation with strangers in a crowded bus, a small elevator, or a supermarket checkout line. But it shouldn't exist at a business meeting, a school lunch break, or the first date with someone special.

Respect someone's "personal space" by standing an appropriate distance away. Your appearance, behavior, and language should draw attention, and standing or sitting very close may actually detract from your actions. Personal space encompasses physical space, mental space, and verbal space, as well as moral and ethical space. Be considerate of others' "comfort zones"; in particular, think about the five senses and try not to make loud noises, wear strong scents, squeeze tightly, or otherwise overwhelm others' senses.

Today, practice keeping just the right physical distance, and use your eyes, smile, and posture to close the gap. Answering a cell phone invades the auditory space of others: excuse yourself and step away if you must take a call, but get your business done quickly and hang up.

Phase 1 | INVITING SUCCESS

MENU

Meal	Recipe	Yield	Calories	P. No.
Breakfast	All-Bran with Apples and Cinnamon	(1 serving)	252	146
Lunch	Macaroni and Cheese a la Francaise	(2 servings)	340	182
Snack	Zucchini Stuffed with Tuna or one peach	(1 serving)	44 (61 for peach)	200
Dinner	Broiled Salmon with Herbs de Provence	(1 serving)	450	160
	Brown Rice Pilaf	(1 serving)		180
Dessert	Have 1 sliced banana with 1 tablespoon chopped walnuts		154	
Total			1240	

EXERCISE

The **Plank:** Our abdominal exercises will be done in two parts. First is the plank position—a great strengthening movement for the deepest ab muscles, which wrap around the whole midsection. When these muscles are toned, your waist becomes thinner, stronger, and tighter.

1. Lie on your stomach, and place your forearms on the ground. Lift your body off the floor on your toes and forearms. Keep your abs tucked in and back straight like a "plank." Relax your shoulders and neck. Remember to breathe throughout. No movement is required—just firm, tucked abs.
2. Hold this position for as long as possible, then return to the floor.
3. Repeat this exercise with this added movement. Keeping your body motionless, lift your straight left leg several inches off the ground, hold for a count of 8—or as long as possible—then lower it back down slowly.
4. Next, lift your right leg off the ground, hold for a count of 8—or as long as possible—then lower it down. Remember to keep abs tucked into back, and shoulders and neck relaxed.

Repeat this until you've worked on each leg 3 times.

The **Reverse Crunch:** For the second part of the exercise, you'll do a reverse crunch, which targets the lower abs.

1. Lie on your back and place your hands on the floor or comfortably behind your head. Bring your slightly bent knees in toward your chest to about 90 degrees, with feet together or crossed.
2. Tuck the abs into the back, and lift the hips off the floor, reaching the legs up towards the ceiling.

3. Lower hips back down as you keep squeezing abs in. Repeat for 10-12 reps or til fatigue.

Note: Keep your head and shoulders flat against the floor at all times. This is a small movement that "packs a big punch." Please use your abs to lift your hips (a small movement) rather than swinging your legs up incorrectly to create momentum. Nice work!

Exercise	Reps	Sets
Plank	Each exercise until	1
Reverse Crunch	fatigued	

FASHION TIP

Accessories are the heart of style. Choose jewelry, watches, shoes, and bags with special care. When in doubt, remember that simplicity is best, and *you* should be the focus of attention, not your apparel.

SELF-CONFIDENCE SKILLS

According to Sigmund Freud, just about everything comes down to sex. Contemporary psychologists believe that this perspective is too simplistic. Nevertheless, it is surprising how many irrational delusions and injurious personal myths have a sexual element. Your assignment today is to study these personal myths and determine if any of them apply to you.

> "If I had a more beautiful body, I would lose control and become sexually promiscuous."
> "If I lose weight, I will gain more attention and my spouse will get jealous and leave me."
> "If I dropped some pounds, I would startle people by walking around naked."

Each of these statements assumes: "If I lost weight something terrible (sexually) would happen." Is there a sexual agenda that keeps you from losing weight? Perhaps there are myths that reflect sexual fears, apprehensions, and discomfort. If so, you could turn harmful personal myths into something more constructive:

> "If I had a more beautiful body, my chances to have close relationships would increase."
> "If I lose weight, I will gain more attention and my spouse will be proud of me."

You need to assess your sexuality, your sexual needs, and your sexual values. Once you have been honest with yourself about your sexual nature, you can enlist sexuality as an ally in adhering to your weigh-loss program.

Phase 1 | INVITING SUCCESS

MENU

Meal	Recipe	Yield	Calories	P. No.
Breakfast	Oatmeal with Raisins and Berries	(1 serving)	221	149
Lunch	Mushroom and Barley Soup	(2 servings)	514	184
Snack	Pear and Almond Bruschetta	(1 serving)	94	199
Dinner	Turkey Breast with Sage	(1 serving)	341	171
Dessert	Chop 1 apple, top with 2 tablespoons slivered almonds, sprinkle with $1/4$ teaspoon ground cinnamon and $1/2$ teaspoon brown sugar. Heat in the microwave for 60 to 90 seconds.		188	
Total			1358	

EXERCISE

This week we will begin to assemble your workout from the individual exercises you learned last week. We'll be doing this very gradually so you can concentrate on form, breathing, and accuracy. You may need to refer back to the previous week's instructions initially, but you'll catch on quickly to the routine before we move up to more challenging levels.

Today, begin with the **squats** and do as many as possible until you are fatigued. Please feel free to use a couch or chair as a marker (not for support) to develop your balance and security with this exercise.

Next, it's on to **push-ups**. Do 1 set of 12, or as many as possible.

Last, move on to your abdominal exercises. First do the **plank**, lifting and holding until fatigued; and then the plank with leg lifts—as many as you can for each leg—with 8 being a good goal for each leg. Then do the **reverse crunch** for 12 reps or until fatigued. You're on your way!

Exercise	Reps/Counts	Sets
Squats	12	1
Push-Ups	12	1

Plank	As long as you can, then 8 leg lifts on each side	1 and 1
Reverse Crunch	12	1

HAIR TIP

Today we will focus on an annoying but very common hair problem: dandruff. Dandruff is your scalp's way of telling you it needs attention and needs to be healed. Technically it's an overabundance of dead skin cells that fall off the scalp. We all know what it looks like: red, irritated, and flaky. The treatment is simple; use a shampoo containing magnesium sulfate as a healing agent to replenish the scalp. Usually, dandruff shampoos are matched with a conditioner, which you can use if necessary. Make sure that you use the appropriate hair products if you have this condition.

INTERPERSONAL SKILLS

Jealousy is one of the least desirable of all human emotions: Shakespeare called it "a green-eyed monster." The better you look, the more socially graceful you are and the greater your achievements, the more likely it is that some acquaintances will feel threatened, inferior, and perhaps hostile.

Incapable of achieving their own life goals, jealous individuals use put-downs, gossip and greed to cope with low self-esteem and lack of accomplishment. But name-calling and envious arrogance have never transformed an underachiever into the center of attention. Jealousy is simply a waste of time and energy.

Accept jealousy as a rite of passage as you continue to improve your appearance and popularity. Pointing out someone else's flaws doesn't automatically make you a better person. Let jealous people live in their own world by their own standards. Figure out who you are, what you want, and how to improve what you don't like. Only compete with yourself.

Turn jealousy around by paying special attention to the person who is jealous. Ignore the jealousy. Sometimes that person just wants to be acknowledged. Remember to give compliments freely to others. Everyone likes to be appreciated and noticed; however, be careful with your delivery of compliments. Give them sincerely so that you do not appear disingenuous.

Phase 1 | INVITING SUCCESS

MENU

Meal	Recipe	Yield	Calories	P. No.
Breakfast	Poached Eggs over Spinach	(1 serving)	246	154
Lunch	Pumpkin Soup and Pepitas	(2 servings)	356	186
Snack	Mix 6 ounces low-fat plain yogurt with 2 teaspoons dried blueberries or raisins		125	
Dinner	Trout with Horseradish	(1 serving)	263	162
	Green Beans with Mushrooms	(1 serving)	94	179
Dessert	Thin Apple Tart	(1 serving)	160	205
Total			1244	

EXERCISE

Today we are going to do two other exercises that you learned last week. First up are **back rows,** using light weights. You're going to do 12, lifting both arms simultaneously—but remember: "the back is the boss" so squeeze your back first, then lift your arms. Do 2 sets of 12 with excellent form to a count of 2-up-and-4-down, and make sure you're breathing correctly: exhale when you lift, inhale when you return your arms to the starting position.

Lunges are next, and don't hesitate to refer to last week's detailed descriptions to remind yourself of the perfect form. Start with the left leg and do 12 reps, then switch to the right leg for another 12. Take a few moments to catch your breath, and then repeat this entire set once.

Last, and certainly not least, you're going to finish with your abdominal exercises, exactly the same as yesterday (and tomorrow, if you're wondering). Do 3 sets of **plank** position lifts on each leg, then 3 sets of **reverse crunches.** Bravo!

Exercise	Reps/Counts	Sets
Back Row	12	1
Lunge	12 left leg / 12 right leg	1
Plank	Hold until fatigued, then 8 leg lifts on each side	1
Reverse Crunch	As many as possible	1

GROOMING TIP

What type of moisturizer do you need for your skin type? The easiest way to begin is to look for moisturizer labeled for your skin type.

Good ingredients for normal to dry skin include peptides, and you can try a serum if you're skin is extremely dry. Note that creams are heavier, and lotions are lighter.

Even oily skin needs moisturizer! Look for an oil-free moisturizer. And all skin types should be sure not to overdo it—just a dime-sized amount should suffice.

SELF-CONFIDENCE SKILLS

Meditative practices can reduce stress, sharpen mental focus, facilitate problem solving, and enhance your spiritual life. They can also help you lose weight.

Many people think that meditation requires that they sit still. But this is not the only way to meditate, simply the best known. Meditation is the ability to deliberately regulate your attention so that you are living entirely in the moment. You can do this while sitting on a pillow in the famous "lotus position" with your legs crossed and "clearing your mind." But you can also do this by sitting in a comfortable chair.

If you would like to give meditation a try, a simple way to start the process is to sit still and repeat a short word such as "one," "love," or "peace" for about twenty minutes. Or focus on a simple design such as a circle (called a "mandala" in some spiritual traditions). If your mind starts to wander, bring it back to the circle and maintain your focus.

Another popular approach is "mindfulness meditation." People who practice this type of meditation spend some time each day being attentive or "mindful" to thoughts that are part of their "mind chatter"; being mindful is an excellent way to detect and release destructive personal myths and lessen daily stress.

Phase 1 | INVITING SUCCESS

MENU

Meal	Recipe	Yield	Calories	P. No.
Breakfast	Muesli with Peach and Almond	(1 serving)	211	147
Lunch	Four Bean Salad	(1 serving)	245	193
Snack	Have $1/_4$ cup whole-milk ricotta cheese mixed with 1 tablespoon apricot preserves and $1/_4$ teaspoon pure almond extract; stir well to combine. Add 2 chopped fresh or canned (juice or water packed) apricots		140	
Dinner	Tuscan Beef Stew	(1 serving)	434	172
Dessert	Winter Fruit Salad	(1 serving)	135	TK
Total			1165	

EXERCISE

It's time to move on to our other two exercises, so let's start with **shoulder presses**. Using your light weights, press up slowly and carefully, 2-up-4-down, then lower your palms back to shoulder level. Aim for 12 times.

Next are **one-arm rows**. Aim for one set.

Our concluding exercise today is once again abdominals, first the **plank**, then the **reverse crunches**, exactly the same way as yesterday. Do a good job—it will show and you'll thank me later.

Exercise	Reps/Counts	Sets
Shoulder Press	12	2
One-Arm Row	Aim for 12 with each arm	2
Plank	15 seconds, then 8 leg lifts on each side	1
Reverse Crunch	12	1

Phase 1 | INVITING SUCCESS

FASHION TIP

Plan ahead: There is no need to tear through your closet in the morning looking for an outfit. Before you go to bed tonight, try on different combinations of colors, fabrics and styles. This will help to prevent a possible fashion faux pas. Make sure all clothing is neatly pressed and ready to wear.

INTERPERSONAL SKILLS

Being late doesn't just cause you to miss a train, a movie, or a dentist appointment. It also makes you appear rude, careless, and disorganized. Being late may also be viewed as extremely selfish behavior, as if only your own schedule is important. Other people's time is just as important as yours. You show a lack of respect to others when you are late. If you are late, apologize profusely and immediately.

Plan your daily activities well in advance and allow yourself extra time to get to each location, especially in big cities like New York. By being on time, you will start off your meeting, meal, or date in the best possible way.

Phase 1 | INVITING SUCCESS

MENU

Meal	Recipe	Yield	Calories	P. No.
Breakfast	All-Bran with Apples and Cinnamon	(1 serving)	252	146
Lunch	Bean Soup	(2 servings)	396	187
Snack	Have 2 tablespoons sunflower seeds and 1 tablespoon dried blueberries		127	
Dinner	Sea Bass with Mango Coulis		329	162
Dessert	Have 1 sliced banana with 1 tablespoon chopped walnuts		154	
Total			1258	

EXERCISE

Today we'll be doing different groupings of the exercises—a little more challenging but still easy enough to allow you to concentrate on your form and breathing.

Here's the order of the exercises, to be done with the same number of reps and sets as previously: **squats**, **push-ups**, **back rows**, **plank**, and **reverse crunches**. Don't forget to breathe correctly and don't forget to check yourself out in a mirror to make sure your form is right.

Exercise	Reps/Counts	Sets
Squats	12	1
Push-Ups	12	1
Back Row	12	2
Plank	15 seconds, then 8 leg lifts on each side	2
Reverse Crunch	12	2

HAIR TIP

Oily hair is a problem for many people. Here is an example of where the cleansing process is really important. Use a shampoo and conditioner that closes the cuticle. Also, beware of using the wrong products. You don't want to use any serums or polishes that bring out or draw attention to the oils in your hair. Be sure these products are light in feel in order to provide shine, but not weight down hair.

Static in hair presents a different problem, but the solution is easy: a light spritz of hair spray can tame static-ridden hair.

What is the solution for split ends? Getting your hair cut frequently will help keep your ends healthy. Brushing your hair properly is also very important. It's best to brush from the bottom of your hair to the root so you work through all the tangles. This will help your hair experience less breakage, thus fewer split ends. You can also try a strengthener, which is made to close the hair cuticle so that split ends aren't visible. It also locks in volume and shine, and will strengthen the hair over time.

SELF-CONFIDENCE SKILLS

If you don't like the idea of meditating, all is not lost. You can live in the moment by engaging in a "flow" experience. Flow usually happens when you are actively involved in a task that stretches and expands your physical and mental abilities. As a result, you don't think of the past, you don't think of the future, you simply focus on the task itself, whether climbing a mountain, playing a game (such as chess or crossword puzzles), or having sex.

How does meditation differ from flow? Meditation is deliberate. You make a decision to start meditating and set a time aside for the activity. Meditation requires practice, and many people attend a class or receive personalized instruction from a master meditator. Flow sneaks up on you; it often happens accidentally, but once you have had the experience you usually want to have it again. You cannot tell yourself to flow; you simply initiate an activity where flow may occur. For example, you may find yourself "flowing" while dancing or while cleaning vegetables. You will be so focused on the dance steps or on scrubbing the carrots that you won't think of food.

Learn to enjoy every bite of food while you are eating. If you bring the skills of meditation or the flow experience to your weight loss program, you will find yourself eating less but enjoying it more.

Phase 1 | INVITING SUCCESS

MENU

Meal	Recipe	Yield	Calories	P. No.
Breakfast	Homemade Granola with Pumpkin Yogurt	(1 serving)	313	148
Lunch	Chicken Salad with Fruit	(1 serving)	376	194
Snack	Zucchini Stuffed with Tuna or 1/2 pink/red grapefruit	(2 servings)	88 53	200
Dinner	Turkey Breast with Sage	(1 serving)	341	171
Dessert	Have 2 sliced fresh peaches topped with 1 tablespoon each chopped walnuts and and slivered almonds		178	
Total			1296	

EXERCISE

Today we'll be doing a different group of the exercises, once again with the same number of reps and sets you've done previously: **lunges**, **shoulder presses**, **one-arm rows**, **plank**, and **reverse crunches**. Don't be afraid to refer back to the previous instructions to keep your form perfect and your breathing patterns correct.

Exercise	Reps/Counts	Sets
Lunge	12 left leg / 12 right leg	2
Shoulder Press	12	2
One-Arm Row	12 with each arm	2
Plank	15 seconds, then 8 leg lifts on each side	2
Reverse Crunch	12	2

GROOMING TIP

A facial scrub or mask can be an enhancing treatment if used appropriately. The type and frequency of use depend on your skin type. If you have oily skin, you can exfoliate almost daily, using a mask or scrub that draws oil out of the skin. If you have sensitive skin, exfoliate only once a week. If you have dry skin, use a mask that can hydrate skin.

A facial is a way of deep cleansing the skin in a way we can't do on our own. The facials of yesteryear are no longer good. Peels and laser treatment are aggressive and state-of-the-art.

INTERPERSONAL SKILLS

"Less is more" in matters of weight, fashion, interior decorating, and even human speech. Today you'll learn a secret that the conversationalists have all mastered: choose your words carefully and edit your remarks.

Most people have a tendency to talk too much, whether about pleasurable subjects or in heated arguments. Unfortunately, once an unkind remark is spoken, it cannot become unspoken, erased, deleted, or retracted gracefully. Never get yourself into a situation where your words run ahead of your thoughts and poison a personal or business relationship.

For this reason, keep an imaginary pair of scissors in your mind when you talk with your friends, family, teachers, co-workers, new acquaintances, or even strangers. If your next sentence contains negativity, insulting words, or unnecessarily controversial material, use the "scissors" to snip the sentence.

Be sure you consider whom you are speaking to: never discuss topics that may make people uncomfortable or embarrassed. And keep in mind that when you speak to people, how they "hear" the meaning is perhaps more important than what you say.

Phase 1 | INVITING SUCCESS

MENU

Meal	Recipe	Yield	Calories	P. No.
Breakfast	Sweet Bell Pepper and Spinach Omelet	(1 serving)	244	152
Lunch	Tom Soup	(1 serving)	343	188
Snack	Have $\frac{1}{2}$ cup cubed honeydew topped with 1 tablespoon chopped walnuts		113	
Dinner	Codfish with Ratatouille	(1 serving)	273	163
	Brown Rice Pilaf	(1 serving)	134	180
Dessert	Thin Apple Tart	(1 serving)	160	205
Total			1267	

EXERCISE

Once again, we're going to do three exercises followed by abdominals, and today those three are **squats**, **push-ups**, and **back rows**—concluding with **plank** and **reverse crunches**, as always. Are you getting the hang of this? Wait until you see the results!

Exercise	Reps/Counts	Sets
Squats	12	2
Push-Ups	12	2
Back Row	12	2
Plank	15 seconds, then 8 leg lifts on each side	2
Reverse Crunch	12	2

Phase 1 | INVITING SUCCESS

FASHION TIP

Layering clothing is a perfect way to create a sharp, flattering look, so spruce up a traditional button-down shirt with an interesting vest, sweater or jacket. Experiment with different materials, mixing velvet with cotton or silk, or matching a sheer shirt with a solid vest or jacket.

Practice mixing and matching at home, and when in doubt, ask for advice from a trusted source.

SELF-CONFIDENCE SKILLS

I'm sure you've heard of programs that help alcoholics and drug users recover from their addictions. Did you ever think that overeating could be a substitute addiction? It is not uncommon for people to stop smoking and start gorging themselves with food. And it can happen the other way around as well. People can lose weight but get hooked on drugs—they have simply exchanged one addiction for another.

This illustrates an important principle of human psychology: People are usually not addicted to a substance; they are addicted to the feelings that these substances evoke. They can also be slaves to personal myths, for example:

"I look really cool smoking cigarettes."

"A three-martini luncheon is necessary to close a business deal."

"I am such a loser that my addiction is simply proof that I am a no-good failure in life."

But by understanding destructive personal myths, downbeat body images, and negative self-concepts, you can stop your descent down the addictive path. So your activity today is to take a careful look at your life to see if you are prone to addictive behavior.

For example, you may find yourself neglecting your work to play a video game. Some people won't let a day go by without their video game "fix," or without their text-messaging gossip or without buying a lottery ticket. Others may decide to have one piece of candy and before they know it they have consumed the entire box. Or at night, a "midnight snack" of a piece of pie becomes an excuse to finish the entire pie.

Phase 1 | INVITING SUCCESS

MENU

Meal	Recipe	Yield	Calories	P. No.
Breakfast	Buckwheat Crêpes with Salmon	(1 serving)	181	150
Lunch	Salade Niçoise au Citron	(1 serving)	489	195
Snack	Dip 7 cherry tomatoes in 1 tablespoon olive tapenade		97	
Dinner	Lamb Chops Roman Style	(1 serving)	322	173
	Broccoli with Parmesan	(1 serving)	189	175
Dessert	Winter Fruit Salad	(1 serving)	135	201
Total			1413	

EXERCISE

Let's finish off the week in grand fashion with another triad of exercises you've already mastered: **lunges**, **shoulder presses**, and **one-arm rows**. You'll finish up with **plank** and **reverse crunches** exercises, everyone's favorite. Congratulations: you're on your way to a more glamorous tomorrow!

Exercise	Reps/Counts	Sets
Lunge	12 left leg / 12 right leg	2
Shoulder Press	12	2
One-Arm Row	12 with each arm	2
Plank	15 seconds, then 8 leg lifts on each side	2
Reverse Crunch	12	2

HAIR TIP

Changing your hair color can be an exciting and creative experience. This is not a modern invention, since many plant-derived dyes have been used for thousands of years. What is right for you? It really just depends on what you like, and what works for your skin tone and features (eye color, brow color). When you work with a colorist, the two of you will find a color that will complement you completely.

Sometimes the very opposite of your natural color makes the best and most appealing look. Don't be afraid to try something new. You can either have a single-process hair color or try highlights.

Ever think of going blond? You can see how you would look simply by trying on a wig. Experiment with different shades of blond, too: dirty blond, strawberry blond, platinum blond. There is no risk involved, and if you don't like what you see, take it off.

Gray hair needs to match a certain image. Who looks good with gray hair? Gray hair looks good on a woman with confidence. It works well with a chic bob.

On the other hand, highlights are right for everyone. How many do you want? How light do you want to go? Do you want subtle, severe, or chunky highlights? Your colorist will be able to guide you.

INTERPERSONAL SKILLS

Children are taught to say "Thank you" in their earliest years. It's part of their limited vocabulary when starting to communicate with their parents, relatives, and caretakers. In fact, it's probably the first "social skill" that anyone learns.

How well have you remembered this lesson? Did you say "Thank you" at every possible opportunity today? If not, you've already started out your day at a disadvantage.

"Thank you" is a very powerful expression. You cannot say it too often. It is a way of showing respect, of letting people know that you are appreciative, and that you value their feelings as much as you value your own. Saying "Thank you" lets others know that you are not above them and do not believe yourself to be.

Because the words are so powerful, never say "Thank you" and not mean it. This is disrespectful and rude, and you might as well not say it at all. You must be sincere; people can read your true feelings in your eyes and body language, so focus on these words when you say them with the right inflection and emphasis.

"Thank you" affords an opportunity for a repeat performance: think of it as "Let's do this again" and say it with a smile.

Phase 1 | INVITING SUCCESS

PREPARING FOR GREATNESS

Phase 2

MENU

Meal	Recipe	Yield	Calories	P. No.
Breakfast	Orange Wheat Muffin	(1 serving)	202	151
Lunch	Lentil Soup with Ground Turkey	(1 serving)	262	189
Snack	Dip 1 sliced orange bell pepper in dressing of 2 teaspoons olive oil, 1 teaspoon of chopped fresh herbs (such as dill and basil), and 1 tablespoon balsamic vinegar		111	
Dinner	Shrimp Scampi	(1 serving)	496	164
Dessert	Have 1 sliced banana with 1 tablespoon chopped walnuts		154	TK
Total			1225	

EXERCISE

Let's start to put it all together. Today's sequence of exercises is as follows: **squats, push-ups, back rows, lunges, plank**, and **reverse crunches**. Keep the number of sets and repetitions the same as you have done in the previous weeks. When you've finished the abdominals, you're done for the day.

Exercise	Reps/Counts	Sets
Squats	12	2
Push-Ups	12	2
Back Row	12	2
Lunge	12 left leg / 12 right leg	2
Plank	20 seconds, then 8 leg lifts on each side	2
Reverse Crunch	12	2

GROOMING TIP

Now let's focus on choosing your colors. Is there a one-size-fits-all formula? No, it's rhyme and reason, trial and error. But always think about how your makeup matches what you're wearing. The general rules have changed drastically over the years but in general, makeup is an accessory to a wardrobe.

The most important first step is to get your skin tone right. If you burn easily, you're probably fair and have a ruddy complexion (your skin has redness). Skin that tans easily is usually medium to olive to dark toned. If you have a ruddy complexion, do not use hot pink. If you have a sallow face, don't wear yellow (coral) but more pink. The proper lipstick can help to balance your skin tone.

SELF-CONFIDENCE SKILLS

Today is the day to focus on "feedback," the information that is "fed back" to you as a result of both external and internal cues. A bathroom scale gives you external feedback, and positive physical feelings provide internal feedback.

When other people compliment your "new look," the feedback is both external and internal. The external feedback comes from your friends and associates; the internal feedback is the positive mood that results from their observations.

Expect some negativity from people who are jealous or from those who simply can not accommodate the changes you are making. Let complimentary comments serve as positive feedback. As for the negative remarks, remember that they usually reflect the personal myths of people who deliver them.

Of course, the most important feedback comes from yourself. If nobody notices your weight loss and you don't receive well-deserved compliments, remember that internal feedback is more important than external feedback. If you are honest with yourself, you will know quite well if you have been succeeding. Your self-confidence will soar if you are making progress and this will set you up to make even greater advancements in the future.

MENU

Meal	Recipe	Yield	Calories	P. No.
Breakfast	Country Frittata	(1 serving)	230	153
Lunch	Salmon and Asparagus Salad	(1 serving)	293	196
Snack	Have 2 tablespoons sunflower seeds and 1 tablespoon dried blueberries		127	
Dinner	Chicken Cacciatora	(1 serving)	489	168
Dessert	Chop 1 apple, top with 2 tablespoons slivered almonds, sprinkle with $1/4$ teaspoon ground cinnamon and $1/2$ teaspoon brown sugar. Heat in the microwave for 60 to 90 seconds.		188	TK
Total			1327	

EXERCISE

Here comes another sequence of exercises as we slowly but surely get your bod in great shape: **back rows**, **lunges**, **shoulder presses**, **one-arm rows**, and **abdominals**. Go to it!

You will not achieve the same level of progress with each of the components of your workout program; some parts may take longer to master. Be patient, and be strong!

Exercise	Reps/Counts	Sets
Back Row	12	2
Lunge	2 left leg / 12 right leg	2
Shoulder Press	12	2
One-Arm Row	12 with each arm	2
Plank	20 seconds, then 8 leg lifts on each side	2
Reverse Crunch	12	2

FASHION TIP

Now that you are an expert at mixing and matching colors and patterns, try experimenting with different materials. Mixing shades of cream in wool, silk, and cotton makes for a fantastic look.

INTERPERSONAL SKILLS

If you think you're already a master of interpersonal relations, consider this: how diverse are the people you interact with every day? It's easy to befriend and converse with others just like yourself. Are you equally skilled with those of a different background?

Throughout your life, you will meet, get to know, and be judged by people whose interests, philosophy, family history, and appearance are unlike your own. Therefore, you need to become comfortable with a wide range of individuals.

Challenge yourself today by having a friendly talk with someone quite different from your usual group of friends. Don't be exclusive, be inclusive. You need not change your style of speech, dress, or behavior. Using empathetic language, good eye contact, warm smiles and minimal gestures, and reach out to someone new.

Give everyone a chance to know you and show respect: you will become a more caring person if you take the time and interest to learn about others and their cultures.

Phase 2 | PREPARING FOR GREATNESS

PREPARING FOR GREATNESS

Phase 2

MENU

Meal	Recipe	Yield	Calories	P. No.
Breakfast	Oatmeal with Raisins and Berries	(1 serving)	221	149
Lunch	Chicken Salad with Fruit	(1 serving)	376	194
Snack	Mix 6 ounces low-fat plain yogurt with 2 teaspoons dried blueberries or raisins		125	
Dinner	Tuna Provençal	(1 serving)	328	155
Dessert	Thin Apple Tart ½ pink or red grapefruit	(1 serving)	160 53	205
Total			1210	

EXERCISE

Today is a "rest" day—no resistance training. Your muscles need time to recover. However it's a great idea to take a brisk walk or put music on and dance around the house. You are building an "exercise habit" so enjoy some type of recreational physical activity at your allotted exercise time every day. Try 50 jumping jacks, or walk up and down the stairs several times. Mix it up—be creative!

HAIR TIP

Despite what you might think, there is such a thing as overloading one's hair with products. This is especially true if you have fine or limp hair and you saturate it with conditioner or a volumizer. You will end up making your hair look greasy and weighing it down. On the other hand, products with alcohol will cause your hair to dry out. Even too much hairspray can cause build up, which is not good for your hair. It will make it look dull and unhealthy. The message is: A little bit of product can go a long way.

By the way, to protect your hair while sleeping, use a silk pillowcase; it's soft and will help prevent tangles.

SELF-CONFIDENCE SKILLS

Today, you're going to work on the vocal component of social skills and start to turn yourself into a "smooth operator." Many people don't recognize the hesitations or standoffishness in their own conversations. Sexy, magnetic, charismatic individuals make every word and inflection count for something, even when they are speaking on the telephone.

Let's try a simple role-playing exercise. Repeat after me: "Hi, there! You look like the person of my dreams, and I'd love to get to know you much better." Now, say it out loud, slowly and somewhat seductively to an imaginary Brad Pitt or Angelina Jolie. Do you need a visual aid? Speak to a photograph in a fan magazine or to yourself in the mirror, pretending you're the object of interest. Be sure your smile, your posture, and your gestures match the allure in your voice.

After a few practice sessions, you'll notice that the tone of your voice has changed to match the task at hand. When you have these few lines down perfectly, simply say only the first two words, "Hi there," leaving off the rest. Invest those two words with as much charm as possible. And now comes the next part of your assignment. Greet everyone today with those words the same way you "spoke" to that movie star.

If you think you need a little reminding, practice the entire greeting again (in your mind, or out loud somewhere where no one can hear you). You may never sound like George Clooney or Kathleen Turner, just an ultra-sensuous version of yourself. You'll be pleased at the results of simply learning how to say "hello" in a much more enticing way. And this feedback will improve your performance the next time that you greet someone!

Phase 1 | PREPARING FOR GREATNESS

Phase 2

MENU

Meal	Recipe	Yield	Calories	P. No.
v **Breakfast**	Poached Eggs over Spinach	(1 serving)	246	154
Lunch	Salad Niçoise au Citron	(1 serving)	489	195
Snack	Dip 10 baby carrots in 1 tablespoon tapenade, or 1 peach		110 61	
Dinner	Chicken au Citron	(1 serving)	245	167
	Zucchini and Bell Peppers with Pine Nuts	(1 serving)	117	176
Dessert	Winter Fruit Salad	(1 serving)	135	201
Total			1342	

EXERCISE

At the risk of sounding repetitious (but definitely for results you will love), we are going to perform the exact sequence we did three days ago. Today's exercises are as follows: **squats, push-ups, back rows, lunges,** and **abdominals.** Keep the number of sets and repetitions the same as you have done in the previous weeks. When you've finished the abdominals, you're done for the day.

Exercise	Reps/Counts	Sets
Squats	12	2
Push-Ups	12	2
Back Row	12	2
Lunge	12 left leg / 12 right leg	2
Plank	20 seconds, then 3 leg lifts on each side	2
Reverse Crunch	12	2

GROOMING TIP

Let's clear up some misconceptions about foundation today. Experts are sometimes asked if one can use foundation to change skin color. What's the answer? You can but you shouldn't. Foundation should match your color and balance some imperfections. Use a finishing powder but first even out the canvas with a foundation. It should blend with your skin.

Another misconception is that we can test foundation or concealer color on the hands. This is not the way to do it. The wrist is completely different from your face. Test the color on a clean face (or cheek or jaw line). Then take a mirror and look in daylight. Don't look in department store light or you might buy the wrong color.

Remember, foundation should end at your jaw line. If it's the right match, there's no need to blend it down along your neck.

INTERPERSONAL SKILLS

Shaking someone's hand may not seem complex to you, but there's a right and a wrong way to do it. You can radiate confidence, warmth, and hospitality with this simple gesture.

Skillful practitioners of this initial attempt at bonding know two things: you can't get too close and you can't be too far. Keep an appropriate distance and use your eyes and smile to close the distance between you and the other individual. Your facial expression and body language are important parts of a handshake.

Use the same force you would need to squeeze a pillow. Guys: an overly firm handshake appears insincere. Ladies: shake a hand firmly while looking the person in the eyes.

Practice an imaginary handshake in the mirror today. Look at yourself: make sure that you would want to meet the person in the mirror. When you get the posture and the facial expression right, practice this with at least three different people and watch their reactions. If politicians of all persuasions can master this skill, so can you!

Phase 2 | PREPARING FOR GREATNESS

PREPARING FOR GREATNESS

Phase 2

MENU

Meal	Recipe	Yield	Calories	P. No.
Breakfast	Buckwheat Crêpes with Salmon	(1 serving)	181	150
Lunch	Mushrooms and Barley Soup	(2 servings)	514	184
Snack	Have 1/2 cup cubed honeydew topped with 1 tablespoon chopped walnuts		113	
Dinner	Broiled Tuna with Tarragon Sauce	(1 serving)	264	157
	Brown Rice Pilaf	(1 serving)	134	180
Dessert	1/2 pink or red grapefruit		53	
Total			1259	

EXERCISE

It's time for another sequence of exercises, the exact same ones you did so well three days ago: **back rows**, **lunges**, **shoulder presses**, **one-arm rows**, **plank**, and **reverse crunches**. Go to it again!

Exercise	Reps/Counts	Sets
Back Row	12	2
Lunge	12 left leg / 12 right leg	2
Shoulder Press	12	2
One-Arm Row	12 with each arm	2
Plank	20 seconds, then 8 leg lifts on each side	2
Reverse Crunch	12	2

FASHION TIP

Check out your local vintage clothing store. You can often find incredible deals on fashionable and impeccably-made pieces of clothing. Examine each item carefully and thoroughly in bright daylight to ensure that it is in good condition and that none of the colors have faded.

SELF-CONFIDENCE SKILLS

Most people start to walk when they are approximately one year old, learning the basics of balance and forward momentum. A baby receives praise when he or she learns how to walk, and that confidence is expressed in "walking tall" as the years go by. However, "walking tall" is not just a reflection of your self-confidence; it's also a way of developing confidence and adding this attitude to your self-concept. Today, you're going to see how.

When you're outdoors today, watch a few other people walking down the street. Ignore those with bad posture, splayed feet, swaying bodies, pot bellies, and dangling arms. Pick out someone athletic, a businessman discussing a project, or someone who might be an actress or a model. At a distance, follow the pace and try to copy the body language. After a minute, turn around and do the same with someone else while walking in the opposite direction. This is another form of role-playing, but this time you have a model to follow.

As you mimic these types, observe what happens in your imagination. You have become just a little bit like them, even though it is temporary. This reaction is typical of role-playing. If you have done your task well, a bit of the person you role played will stay with you for a while.

Once you find a role that seems to match your skills and your abilities, go a bit deeper. What are you feeling and thinking when you imitate another person's body language, posture, and physical movements? The body and mind work together, and role-playing has an external component as well as an internal component. If you want to incorporate them into your own repertoire, simply rehearse them as you would if you were preparing for a part in a play, film, or television series. And you really are preparing, except that the big production number is your new way of living.

Phase 2 | PREPARING FOR GREATNESS

MENU

Meal	Recipe	Yield	Calories	P. No.
Breakfast	Sweet Bell Pepper and Spinach Omelet	(1 serving)	224	152
Lunch	Pasta with Vegetables and Sundried Tomatoes	(1 serving)	347	181
Snack	Zucchini Stuffed with Tuna,	(2 servings)	88	200
	or 1 plum		30	
Dinner	Chicken Cacciatora	(1 serving)	489	168
Dessert	Chocolate Square with Raspberry Coulis	(1 serving)	138	203
Total			1242	

EXERCISE

Another day off! How lucky can you get? Take advantage of this generous offer, but for bonus points, take a 20-minute brisk walk again and/or experiment with lying on the floor and stretching in every direction like a cat—ahhh!

HAIR TIP

You need to have a haircut every six to eight weeks, regardless of the color, length, or texture of your hair. Please don't trim your own hair. The cost saving is not worth it because you cannot perform this task evenly and correctly yourself.

When it comes to coloring, the rules are similar. Depending on what you need done, you should color your hair about every six weeks to keep your color looking fresh and natural. If you are touching up gray hairs you might have to go every three to four weeks.

Women often ask which the easiest up-do is: the French twist; all you have to do is make a ponytail, twist, and pin it up.

INTERPERSONAL SKILLS

Words are a way of getting your message to other people, no matter what the topic is—romance, homework, or the weather.

But let's not concern ourselves today with what you're saying; let's focus on how it sounds. If the sound of your voice is a turnoff, nothing else will work. How you are heard and perceived is often much more important than what you are saying, since human communication always includes a speaker and a listener.

Modulate your voice and try to speak softly. Use inflection when you talk, not volume. Don't "drown out" others' words by speaking over them.

Today try to listen to yourself as you speak with others. Are you pronouncing every letter and syllable? Is your voice shrill and harsh or velvet smooth and alluring? Are you speaking too loudly to someone just a few feet away?

Practice proper vocal control today. Concentrate on diction, volume, clarity, speed, and tone, not content. Focus as well on your hands, eyes, and mouth when speaking, but not affectedly.

In the theater of life, excellent speech is not merely a technique of communicating; it's a way to become the center of attention.

Phase 2 | PREPARING FOR GREATNESS

PREPARING FOR GREATNESS

Phase 2

MENU

Meal	Recipe	Yield	Calories	P. No.
Breakfast	Muesli with Peach and Almond	(1 serving)	211	147
Lunch	Tom Soup	(1 serving)	343	188
Snack	Have ¼ cup whole-milk ricotta cheese mixed with 1 tablespoon apricot preserves and ¼ teaspoon pure almond extract; stir well to combine. Add 2 chopped fresh or canned (juice or water packed) apricots		140	
Dinner	Salmon a l'Orange	(1 serving)	368	159
Dessert	Thin Apple Tart	(1 serving)	160	205
Total			1222	

EXERCISE

Let's finish the week in grand fashion by truly putting it all together: **squats**, **push-ups**, **back rows**, **lunges**, **shoulder presses**, **one-arm rows**, and **abdominals**. Do one set of each exercise in a "circuit"—then come back and do another circuit. Congratulations—excellent job! Reward yourself with a warm bath full of Epsom salts (regular drugstore variety) and sea salt (from the grocery store—about a cup each) for an extra soothing touch.

Exercise	Reps/Counts	Sets
Squats	12	2
Push-Ups	12	2
Back Row	12	2
Lunge	12 left leg / 12 right leg	2
Shoulder Press	12	2
One-Arm Row	12 with each arm	
Plank	20 seconds, then 8 leg lifts on each side	2
Reverse Crunch	12	2

Do this entire circuit twice!

GROOMING TIP

Experts are often asked how to keep eyeliner, mascara, and lipstick in place. Here are some special tips. After applying eyeliner, dip a Q-tip or makeup sponge into translucent powder. Carefully pat the powder just below the eyeliner line. The powder will prevent the liner from smearing.

When you are applying mascara, don't panic if you blink and some mascara ends up above or below your eye. Instead, wait a few moments until the mascara dries. Then, use a Q-tip to remove the mascara—the mascara should flake right off.

Another trick is to use loose powder to help seal lipstick. Here are words of wisdom from the old days, an old-fashioned trick from the theater. Take a tissue and separate it so that you have one thin layer. Apply lipstick as usual, and then place the thin tissue over your lips. Dip a fluffy powder brush or a rouge brush into translucent loose powder and then coat the tissue that is placed on your lips. A small, unnoticeable dusting of powder will pass through the tissue onto your lips and help seal the lipstick. Finally, blot your lips together.

There are also clear overcoats like lip sealers. They will seal lipstick in place, but because they are alcohol-based, they can sometimes be drying. That's why, for day-long events, I reccomend the old "theater trick" above.

SELF-CONFIDENCE SKILLS

Many of your personal myths may relate to social situations that affect your eating habits. People do not exist in a vacuum. Interactions with other women and men are inevitable. Whether you are a "loner" or a "social butterfly," you can't escape the impact of others. Try to make those interactions serve your healthy lifestyle, not undermine it. Here are some personal myths that can sabotage your best intentions to lose weight and keep it from sneaking back.

"A broken heart can best be mended with a double cheeseburger."

"There is no mood so sour that a fried donut can't turn it into bliss."

"The best medicine for an anxiety attack is a slice of lemon meringue pie."

Take a close look at those personal myths. They imply that a quick food fix will bring relief from a social disaster and the resulting inner turmoil. Myths of this nature negate the value of rational thinking and learned optimism. You can transform your thoughts and feelings by reframing your personal myths. Take a look at these new statements; some may apply directly to you!

"Relationships are risky and love is an unpredictable venture. But nothing ventured, nothing gained! The best way to heal my broken heart is to ask what lesson I can learn while being thankful for the good times that relationship brought my way. Life moves on, and I need to move along with it."

"Moods come and go, but a disagreeable mood can shift more quickly if I shift my attention to my favorite sport, my favorite form of exercise, or some other activity that allows me to flow instead of to curdle."

"It's easy to find interpersonal problems to worry about. But for each faux pas or social error, I can come up with two interactions where I behaved admirably. Apathy and pessimism or activity and optimism represent my choices; I will choose the latter."

Phase 2 | PREPARING FOR GREATNESS

MENU

Meal	Recipe	Yield	Calories	P. No.
Breakfast	Country Frittata	(1 serving)	230	153
Lunch	Spinach and Onion Soup	(2 servings)	394	185
Snack	Pear and Almond Bruschetta	(1 serving)	94	199
	½ pink or red grapefruit		53	
Dinner	Turkey Breast with Sage	(1 serving)	341	171
	Zucchini and Bell Peppers with Pine Nuts	(1 serving)		
Dessert	Acai and Berries Popsicles	(1 serving)	76	202
Total			1188	

EXERCISE

A day of rest—but go outside for a walk, or take a swim or a bike ride . . . or have a freestyle dance-fest to your favorite tune! Twist, anyone?

FASHION TIP

Learn how to go from office to a dinner party in a matter of moments. Women: add dressy pieces of jewelry, elegant shoes, and a clutch purse to a little black dress for an easy and stunning look. Men: put on a more formal shirt and tie and add cufflinks .If you need a quick pick-me-up before your soiree, hit the gym or visit the hairdresser. You will feel energized and confident.

INTERPERSONAL SKILLS

"What's in a name?" Shakespeare asked, and you know the answer: you feel wonderful when someone you've met only once or twice knows your name. Therefore, practice this important skill today on someone else.

Introduce yourself to someone at school, work, or the store today. When you hear his or her name, concentrate on remembering it and repeating it in the next three to four sentences. Also, when meeting someone new, focus on the person and remember some small detail about him or her which will enable you to recall the name later.

Horrors! If you forget a person's name and he or she is approaching you (and your friend Lauren), say "Hi there. You remember my friend Lauren, don't you?" Hopefully, this will allow introductions to proceed smoothly.

However, if you have forgotten someone's name and there is no third person around, you have to simply be honest. Say, "Please tell me your name again. I want to commit it to memory so that I never forget it again." You may also want to add, "Please forgive me, I am simply terrible with names."

Phase 3 | MAKING THE A-LIST

MENU

Meal	Recipe	Yield	Calories	P. No.
Breakfast	Homemade Granola with Pumpkin Yogurt	(1 serving)	313	148
Lunch	Chicken Salad with Fruit	(1 serving)	376	194
Snack	Have 2 tablespoons sunflower seeds and 1 tablespoon dried blueberries		127	
Dinner	Broiled Salmon with Herbs de Provence and Brown Rice Pilaf	(1 serving) (1 serving)	450	160 180
Dessert	Have 1 1/2 cups of mixed berries, raspberries, and blackberries		98	
Total			1487	

EXERCISE

We ended last week with a complete cycle of your seven exercises in two circuits, done one after another with good form and careful attention to breathing. And that's exactly where we're going to start off today. Here's a reminder about the exercises, their sequence, and a few special notes:

Squats: you'll be doing 2 sets of 12.

Push-ups: Also 2 sets of 12, but if this feels too easy, try military push-ups—start in plank position, your body in alignment "in one piece," head straight forward. Don't look up or down. If this is too challenging, try 2 military push-ups, then 10 on your knees.

Back rows: 2 sets of 12 stretching out fully after each set.

Lunges: 12 reps for each leg, done one side at a time, in two sets.

Shoulder presses: do 2 sets, lifting both hand weights 12 times. Rest between sets.

One-arm rows: remember that each set entails alternating your left and right arms for 6 rows each, then 6 rows using both arms. Do 2 sets today, resting in between.

Plank: you'll continue to do these as you have before, lifting each leg for a count of 8 twice, alternating the left and right side.

Reverse crunch: In the second part of the exercise, flat on your back, do 2 sets, keeping your legs as close to the floor as possible.

Exercise	Reps/Counts	Sets
Squats	12	2
Push-Ups	12	2
Back Row	12	2
Lunge	12 left leg / 12 right leg	2
Shoulder Press	12	2
One-Arm Row	12 with each arm	
Plank	30 seconds, then 8 leg lifts on each side	2
Reverse Crunch	12	2

Do this circuit twice.

HAIR TIP

If you have long hair, you will need to develop special techniques for its maintenance. When brushing long hair you should always start at the bottom and work your way up to the root. Be sure to hold on to hair in the middle so as not to break off split ends. By doing this you are detangling your hair so there is less breakage.

It is also important to use a product such as a leave-in conditioner. Every type of hair can benefit from a leave-in conditioner. This will help loosen tangles and knots and help protect your hair so you can comb through it with greater ease. Also use a boar bristle brush.

SELF-CONFIDENCE SKILLS

Eat your meals alone today or with a small group of people.

Did you know that the larger the number of people at a meal, the more food you are likely to consume? Furthermore, you become distracted by conversation and tend not to notice the second or third helping.

Don't let this happen today. Your focus is on savoring your meal, not gossiping or wheeling and dealing financial plans. This is a "slow food" day, not a "fast food" day.

Phase 3 | MAKING THE A-LIST

MENU

Meal	Recipe	Yield	Calories	P. No.
Breakfast	All-Bran with Apples and Cinnamon	(1 serving)	252	146
Lunch	Beet Salad	(1 serving)	278	190
Snack	Have 1 tablespoon dried cranberries or blueberries with 2 tablespoons chopped walnuts		123	
Dinner	Tuscan Beef Stew	(1 serving)	434	172
Dessert	Chocolate Square with Raspberry Coulis	(1 serving)	138	203
Total			1225	

EXERCISE

Your exercise today takes place outdoors. We'll return to our training program tomorrow. Take a brisk walk today for 20 minutes in natural surroundings, if possible, and away from traffic. When the weather's bad, you can walk indoors as a sports facility or a mall, or even march in place at home. Even if you feel like doing floor exercises, it's super-important to stretch your muscles out every few days.

GROOMING TIP

Like most people, you probably enjoy summertime activities including sunbathing. However, as we all know by now, sunbathing is not good for the skin, especially delicate facial skin. Please protect it. It is the most susceptible to the aging process. Use wide-brim hats and umbrellas.

Use sunscreen with SPF 30 or more, even when driving in the car. Always use sunscreen on your face, whether it is applied under or over your foundation. Start with a layer of sunscreen that is SPF 30 or more. This is important because foundation placed on top of sunscreen actually degenerates the sunscreen's SPF, making it less powerful (but, if you apply powder with SPF very last, you don't need to worry).

If you really like the way you look with a tan, bronzer is a great way of mimicking a "sun-kissed" look. Bronzer adds pigment to the skin and gives a healthy glow. Be careful if your skin is fair and use very little—you never want to look like you have a bad fake tan.

INTERPERSONAL SKILLS

Military strategists say that it's sometimes better to lose a battle in order to win the war. In relationships, it's often better to lose (or defuse) an argument rather than jeopardize or actually destroy a friendship. People whose relationships or marriages have lasted many decades have mastered the art of compromise and concession. If you want to preserve your most intimate friendships, you must master this extremely important skill. Moreover, it is also necessary to avoid arguments with classmates, co-workers, and family members.

You can be assertive and polite without resorting to anger and demeaning words. Never raise your voice. Look the person in the eye and allow him/her the courtesy of explaining his/her position. Explain clearly what your expectations are and why you believe the situation needs to be handled in the manner you suggest.

Start with a level playing field. Never assume that you have the right to force your position on others or to acquiesce to someone more forceful than yourself.

Arguments bring out the worst in everyone. There are many ways to defuse an argument: say that you are not comfortable; let the other person win a little; stop insisting that your point of view is correct. Instead of arguing, deal with upsetting issues by resolving them.

Phase 3 | MAKING THE A-LIST

MENU

Meal	Recipe	Yield	Calories	P. No.
Breakfast	Sweet Bell Pepper and Spinach Omelet	(1 serving)	224	152
Lunch	Pumpkin Soup and Pepitas	(2 servings)	356	186
Snack	Have $1/2$ cup cubed honeydew topped with 1 tablespoon chopped walnuts		113	
Dinner	Trout with Horseradish	(1 serving)	263	161
	Green Beans with Mushroom	(1 serving)	94	179
Dessert	Thin Apple Tart or $1/2$ pink or red grapefruit	(1 serving)	160 53	205
Total			1210	

EXERCISE

Welcome back to the exercise (double) circuit. Today we're going to make your squats just a teensy bit more challenging by adding light weights. For additional muscle-building, how about doing 3 sets of 12? Watch your form in the mirror and double-check your breathing pattern, inhaling on the way down, exhaling on the way up.

After squats, the rest of the workout is the same as before: push-ups, back rows, lunges, shoulder presses, one-arm rows, plank, and reverse crunches.

Exercise	Reps/Counts	Sets
Squats	12	3
Push-Ups	12	3
Back Row	12	3
Lunge	12 left leg / 12 right leg	3
Shoulder Press	12	3
One-Arm Row	12 with each arm	3
Plank	30 seconds, then 8 leg lifts on each side	3
Reverse Crunch	12	3

Do this circuit twice.

FASHION TIP

Buy a scarf, shawl or tie that adds a splash of color to a basic outfit. Look for colors that bring out your eyes: intense pink for green eyes, green for blue eyes, orange for brown eyes, blue for gray eyes, and yellow for dark eyes.

SELF-CONFIDENCE SKILLS

Eye contact is not just a means of recognizing your friends and family. It's a powerful social skill, mastered by business executives, politicians, and many of the sexiest people on earth. For them, avoiding eye contact is a message of shame, inferiority, and insecurity. Even if you don't like someone, avoiding eye contact gives that person an edge of superiority, power, and control. Therefore, use your eyes to maximal effect.

By the way, there are some cultural groups where women are discouraged from making direct eye contact with men; a culturally sensitive person will be aware of this and act accordingly. Standing in front of your home mirror, look into your eyes the way a stage hypnotist might. Don't merely look at the whites or the iris (the colorful part) of the eyes. Pretend that you are looking right through the pupils into the back of the eye itself. Don't focus on eyebrows, eyelashes, or eyelids, just the two little black dots that, some say, are the windows into someone's soul.

Then, practice on friends, family, coworkers, strangers, even pets. Every time you face these people (or animals), look right at the pupils of their eyes. There's nothing particularly alluring or romantic about this skill, but when you put it together with everything else, whammo!

When a well-dressed person with a svelte body and an alluring voice looks you directly in the eyes, you might melt, you might be magnetized, or you might get turned on. But you won't ignore the experience, and neither will people whom you greet in this manner.

Phase 3 | MAKING THE A-LIST

MENU

Meal	Recipe	Yield	Calories	P. No.
Breakfast	Orange Wheat Muffin	(1 serving)	202	151
Lunch	Four Bean Salad	(1 serving)	245	193
Snack	Dip 1 sliced orange bell pepper in dressing of 2 teaspoons olive oil, 1 teaspoon of chopped fresh herbs (such as dill and basil), and 1 tablespoon balsamic vinegar		111	TK
Dinner	Turkey Breast with Sage and	(1 serving)	458	171 176
	Zucchini and Bell Peppers with Pine Nuts	(1 serving)		
Dessert	1 peach	(1 serving)	61	
Total			1077	

EXERCISE

"Once more with feeling"—let's repeat the double circuit today, using hand weights throughout squats and the other designated exercises. As you get stronger and fitter, it will be increasingly necessary for you to stretch—but the good news is that stretches and aerobics are a built-in part of this exercise program. Walking on your "days off" is also a great way to stretch. Your muscles will thank you.

Exercise	Reps/Counts	Sets
Squats	12	3
Push-Ups	12	3
Back Row	12	3
Lunge	12 left leg / 12 right leg	3
Shoulder Press	12	3
One-Arm Row	12 with each arm	
Plank	30 seconds, then 8 leg lifts on each side	3
Reverse Crunch	12	3

Do this circuit twice.

HAIR TIP

Hair loss, a hereditary problem, afflicts many women and men. There is no way to stop this type of hair loss—it is not due to stress or overprocessing, or anything external. If you notice your hair loss is speeding up, you should consult a dermatologist. He or she can help you determine what products may help (I do believe some products work quite well.)

INTERPERSONAL SKILLS

The art of social interactions includes the appropriate use of tact. Tact means being careful to avoid accidentally hurting someone's feelings.

Tactful remarks are not lies: they are ways of turning negativity into productive, positive advice and observations. "You didn't win the talent contest tonight, but you're getting better every day." "The team played quite well today, but wait until next week!"

Tactful remarks are not delusions, misinformation, or examples of unrealistic optimism. They allow you to help a friend or family member cope with a current problem and give him or her hope for a pleasant solution. Tact allows you to be comforting and inspiring at the same time. Tact also allows you to move beyond minor errors in behavior, dress, or achievement and emphasize positive progress in the future.

Practice a few tactful remarks today. You are going to need this interpersonal skill very often throughout your life.

Phase 3 | MAKING THE A-LIST

MAKING THE A-LIST | **Phase 3**

MENU

Meal	Recipe	Yield	Calories	P. No.
Breakfast	Homemade Granola with Pumpkin Yogurt	(1 serving)	313	148
Lunch	Bean Soup	(2 servings)	396	187
Snack	Dip 10 baby carrots in 1 tablespoon tapenade		110	
Dinner	Sea Bass with Mango Coulis and	(1 serving)	463	162
	Brown Rice Pilaf		134	180
Dessert	Chocolate Square with Raspberry Coulis	(1 serving)	138	203
Total			1554	

EXERCISE

It's a "rest day" once again, but that really should mean a brisk 20-minute walk. Stretching your legs on non-exercise days prevents lactic acid build-up, which causes muscle aches and cramps.

GROOMING TIP

It's important to know the best way to apply lipstick and which type is right for you. There are three main types of lipstick: matte, gloss, and frost. If your lips tend to be dry, stay away from frost or matte textures, and choose a cream formula instead.

If you have time, start with a lip brush. This will give you more accuracy, and the look as a whole will be more polished and finished. Your lipstick will also last longer.

If you are short on time, lip gloss is a great quick alternative to lipstick. Accuracy is not needed as much during application, and the gloss adds shine.

Here is an easy trick: if lips are thin and you want to make them appear fuller, apply lipstick first, then outline your lips with a lip pencil in a matching color.

SELF-CONFIDENCE SKILLS

It's time to take a bold move forward. You'll need a group of people around you for today's exercise, whether they are classmates, fellow workers, or even strangers at a sporting event.

Who is the best-looking or most dynamic person in the group? Pick whomever you want and get ready to catch his or her attention for just a microsecond.

If you're unsure of what to say, keep it brief. This is not the beginning of a lifelong relationship, just an exercise in building self-confidence. Here are some suggestions: "I hope you're having a nice day." "Our team is really performing well today." "Isn't nature great?" (Of course this last remark depends on the weather). None of these greetings requires a response, and don't feel bad if you don't get one. Today's activity simply asks you to practice talking to someone very handsome, beautiful, or powerful. It's easier than it seems. And what do you have to lose?

When you're ready, go for it. Be aware of the tone of your voice, make perfect eye contact, act as relaxed as possible, and smile as if you had just won an Academy Award, a sports trophy, or an election. That's all you need to do today. Don't attempt a long conversation or wait for an acknowledgement. You're just practicing, and you should feel free to try this out again on another person at another time today. Make sure you pick someone whom you wouldn't think of speaking to under ordinary circumstances.

Try this several times with different people, and by the fourth or fifth try you won't have your initial hesitations. Eventually, perhaps fortuitously, you may even wind up in an actual conversation or even a relationship.

Phase 3 | MAKING THE A-LIST

MENU

Meal	Recipe	Yield	Calories	P. No.
Breakfast	Poached Eggs over Spinach	(1 serving)	246	154
Lunch	Salad Niçoise au Citron	(1 serving)	489	195
Snack	Zucchini Stuffed with Tuna	(1 serving)	44	200
Dinner	Lamb Chops Roman Style	(1 serving)	322	173
	Broccoli with Parmesan	(1 serving)	189	175
Dessert	Acai and Berries Popsicles	(1 serving)	76	202
Total			1366	

EXERCISE

By now you have memorized the entire workout circuit, and part of this can be termed "muscle memory" as well. We'll run through it in its entirety from beginning to end as usual, but don't rush like you're late for an appointment. "Slow and steady wins the race" and for our purposes, this means attention to form, breathing, and a slow pace.

Exercise	Reps/Counts	Sets
Squats	12	3
Push-Ups	12	3
Back Row	12	3
Lunge	12 left leg / 12 right leg	3
Shoulder Press	12	3
One-Arm Row	12 with each arm	3
Plank	30 seconds, then 8 leg lifts on each side	3
Reverse Crunch	12	3

Do this circuit twice.

FASHION TIP

If you are not sure how to begin building your new wardrobe, ask a salesperson at your favorite department store or boutique. He or she will be best able to help you choose flattering styles and sizes.

INTERPERSONAL SKILLS

You might be the greatest speaker amongst your friends, family, schoolmates, coworkers, and community, but it's equally important to know the opposite skill: you've also got to be a great listener.

When someone else "has the floor," do your eyes or thoughts wander? Do you look bored or eager to interrupt? Do you fidget or squirm unless you are the center of attention? Silence is a golden opportunity, and here's how it can "speak" for you.

Instead of monopolizing a conversation, lose yourself in the other person's world and thoughts so that you are able to understand his or her problems, ideas and priorities. Concentrate on facial and bodily expressions that radiate your empathy and concern. Every part of you (mouth, legs, and upper body) needs to be centered on other people when you are listening.

Being a good listener is not merely a form of politeness; it's an important way to bond with others and develop mutual trust and respect. It's also a way for you to learn more about the person you're listening to.

Phase 3 | MAKING THE A-LIST

MENU

Meal	Recipe	Yield	Calories	P. No.
Breakfast	Oatmeal with Raisins and Berries	(1 serving)	221	149
Lunch	Tom Soup	(1 serving)	343	188
Snack	Have ¼ cup whole-milk ricotta cheese mixed with 1 tablespoon apricot preserves and ¼ teaspoon pure almond extract; stir well to combine. Add in 2 chopped fresh or canned (juice or water packed) apricots		140	
Dinner	Codfish with Ratatouille	(1 serving)	273	163
	Brown Rice Pilaf	(1 serving)	134	180
Dessert	Thin Apple Tart or 1 plum	(1 serving)	160 30	205
Total			1271	

EXERCISE

Exercising effectively has many benefits, and you're probably starting to feel some of those: better posture, more energy, better sleep, and even more self-confidence. When you feel stronger, you act stronger!

With that in mind, we're going to run through our dynamic routine today as before, but get ready for some changes in the next few days—in our workout and in your body.

Exercise	Reps/Counts	Sets
Squats	12	3
Push-Ups	12	3
Back Row	12	3
Lunge	12 left leg / 12 right leg	3
Shoulder Press	12	3
One-Arm Row	12 with each arm	3
Plank	30 seconds, then 3 leg lifts on each side	3
Reverse Crunch	12	3

Do this circuit twice.

HAIR TIP

When you go to the hair salon, you will usually have a scalp massage in addition to your shampoo. But don't wait for six weeks for this important scalp therapy. Massage your scalp every day for 10 minutes. A combination of smooth circular motions, alternating between fast and slow, will promote circulation and stimulate energy. Massage circulates the blood flow and feeds the root of your hair follicle.

SELF-CONFIDENCE SKILLS

Contemporary psychologists have found that once people have an income that takes them out of the poverty circle, there is no relationship between how much money they make and how happy they are. On the other hand, positve personal relationships, flow experiences, and the enjoyment of one's thoughts, feelings, and experiences are closely related to reports of "being happy."

In no way does self-regulation interfere with one's enjoyment of food and drink. Indeed, wine-tasters, gourmet chefs, and restaurant critics exert a great amount of discipline to keep their taste buds sensitive so that they can share their delight in food and drink with the general public.

Your assignment today is to visit a restaurant and pretend that you are a food critic who is evaluating the cuisine for an international travel magazine. Take small bites (and sips). Take your time in relishing what you eat and drink. Invent your own "star" system and decide what award to give the restaurant. Then give "stars" to each item that you tasted.

Do not think that you have to finish every dish that you are served. Most restaurants in the United States serve oversized meals, thinking that this will draw and keep customers. If you are truly concerned with food waste, donate money to such organizations as Second Harvest that collect unused food from restaurants at the end of the day and distribute it to the poor and needy.

You will truly deserve some "stars" of your own.

Phase 3 | MAKING THE A-LIST

Phase 3 | MAKING THE A-LIST

MENU

Meal	Recipe	Yield	Calories	P. No.
Breakfast	Country Frittata	(1 serving)	230	153
Lunch	Salad Niçoise au Citron	(1 serving)	489	195
Snack	Spinach and Mozzarella Bruschetta	(1 serving)	55	198
Dinner	Shrimp Scampi	(1 serving)	496	164
Dessert	Have 1 1/2 cups of mixed berries, raspberries, and blackberries		98	
Total			1368	

EXERCISE

Here are some embellishments to your routine. Some may be more challenging for you than others so see which you can do comfortably.

Squats: if you haven't tried these with hand weights, now is a good opportunity. But if you're really up to speed, do a jump in between the squats, about 6 inches in the air.

Push-ups: try to do as many of these in military style, not on the knees, but keep to a goal of 12 reps in 3 sets. Feeling more advanced? Keep your hands closer together, challenging the triceps. Want a further challenge for today or later this week? Elevate your feet on a bed. The slower you do a push-up, the more effective it is, so instead of a normal count (4-2), try 4-4 or even 6-6.

Master these first, then we'll be ready for a few new challenges tomorrow.

Exercise	Reps/Counts	Sets
Squats	12	3
Push-Ups	12	3
Back Row	12	3
Lunge	12 left leg / 12 right leg	3
Shoulder Press	12	3
One-Arm Row	12 with each arm	3
Plank	30 seconds, then 3 leg lifts on each side	3
Reverse Crunch	12	3

Do this circuit twice.

GROOMING TIP

Always use blush to add luminosity and brighten your face. But be aware that blush is not just about adding color; it helps bring out your cheekbones so that your face looks more sculpted.

Start with just a little bit of blush, dipping your brush and tapping off the excess. Make a "fish face." You want to start applying blush near your hairline, lining up your brush with the top part of your ear. Sweep color down to the apple of your cheek. Then, after you apply eyeshadow, use some blush on your eyelids.

Remember: blush does not belong on the tip of your nose, on your chin, or on your forehead!

INTERPERSONAL SKILLS

Having a sense of humor is one of the most important interpersonal skills one can possess. Humor has the power to relax, disarm, and stimulate an audience, even if that audience is only one person.

Look for a way to bring laughter and joy into your conversations, but choose your subjects carefully. Avoid politics, religion, and celebrity gossip; these "hot-button topics" may produce unwanted reactions.

Making fun of other people is counterproductive behavior: the listeners might assume that you may eventually ridicule them too. On the other hand, making fun of yourself can actually be a plus, since it implies humility and self-deprecation.

Everyone likes to laugh, and virtually everyone is attracted to witty, happy, and entertaining people who emanate a feeling of fun and enjoyment of life. Smiles and laughter will make you more approachable . . . and happier too.

Phase 3 | MAKING THE A-LIST

MENU

Meal	Recipe	Yield	Calories	P. No.
Breakfast	Homemade Granola with Pumpkin Yogurt	(1 serving)	313	148
Lunch	Lentil Soup with Ground Turkey	(2 servings)	524	189
Snack	Have $1/2$ cup cubed honeydew topped with 1 tablespoon chopped walnuts		113	
Dinner	Tuna Provencal	(1 serving)	328	155
Dessert	$1/2$ pink or red grapefruit		53	
Total			1331	

EXERCISE

Another rest day, perfect for walking outdoors. Take a brisker pace than usual, and perhaps you can lengthen the duration to 30 or 40 minutes.

FASHION TIP

Now that you are slimming down, begin investing in classic pieces that will form the building blocks of your new wardrobe. Basic items for women include: pant suits, skirts, khakis, knits, cocktail dress; for men: blazer, shirts, polo shirts, black tie. Trendy clothing, while alluring, rarely has a long shelf-life. Instead, invest in classic pieces. Consider it a trend that never goes out of style.

Watch out for trendy garments. You'll wear them a couple of times until they get dated, then banish them to the back of the closet. You don't want to have a museum of clothing. Every article should be stylish, contemporary, and flattering.

SELF-CONFIDENCE SKILLS

Your body image and the impression it creates on others depend a great deal on how you look while you are walking. So today let's focus on improving what people see when you walk into a room.

Ever watch those television variety shows where authors and movie stars make celebrity appearances to publicize their latest books and films? Today, you will be the star, the celebrity that the audience at home and in the studio simply can't wait to see "in person."

Use a mirror at home, a full-length mirror if possible. Leave the room, close the door, and gather your thoughts. Imagine that your "fans" are watching from across the country. Imagine there is a studio audience that has waited for hours in the snow, rain, or heat just to get a glimpse of you.

Now open the door, stand up as tall as possible and walk toward the mirror, then turn gracefully until your full face and body face the mirror. Look right into your own eyes, widening them like you just won an Oscar and smile at yourself.

Practice this role-playing about nine or ten times, until you have your "talk-show" entrance down perfectly. You may exaggerate the part played by your eyes and teeth since this is also the way people will first catch sight of you at a party or family event. And wouldn't it be wonderful if someday someone did this exercise with you in mind?

Phase 3 | MAKING THE A-LIST

MENU

Meal	Recipe	Yield	Calories	P. No.
Breakfast	All-Bran with Apples and Cinnamon	(1 serving)	252	146
Lunch	Salmon and Asparagus Salad	(1 serving)	292	196
Snack	Zucchini Stuffed with Tuna or melon slice	(2 servings)	88 46	200
Dinner	Chicken with Mushrooms	(1 serving)	268	165
	Brown Rice Pilaf	(1 serving)	134	180
Dessert	Chocolate Square with Raspberry Coulis	(1 serving)	138	203
Total			1173	

EXERCISE

Today, we'll be doing our usual circuit, perhaps with the addition of the upgrades you learned yesterday. Here are a few more for the strong and daring amongst us:

Lunges: instead of maintaining the previous form, try this intermediate-level addition: step forward about 2 to 3 feet carefully for each lunge, making sure that your knee is directly over your ankle. Push off the front foot to get back to standing position, and be sure to keep your abs firm.

Shoulder presses: while you do this upper body exercise, stand on one leg while you put the big toe of the opposite foot on the floor. Now you have to balance! Never lock your knees, and check your form out in the mirror.

Keep a mental (or written) note of your progress toward these intermediate-level variations. If you don't get it right this time, wait until your strength and balance have improved.

Exercise	Reps/Counts	Sets
Squats	12	3
Push-Ups	12	3
Back Row	12	3
Lunge	12 left leg / 12 right leg	3

Phase 3 | MAKING THE A-LIST

Shoulder Press	12	3
One-Arm Row	12 with each arm	3
Plank	30 seconds, then	3
	8 leg lifts on each side	
Reverse Crunch	12	3

Do this circuit twice.

HAIR TIP

Summertime weather can affect your hair dramatically. Specifically, humidity will cause your hair to frizz, no matter what type it is. Therefore, use an anti-humectant to calm frizzy hair and flyaways. An anti-humectant will stop the moisture from the environment from getting absorbed into hair (which is what frizz is—hair expanding from moisture).

Use a hair polish or calming serum that will help your hair look sleek and shiny. Then finish with a blast of cold air from your blow-dryer to seal the deal.

INTERPERSONAL SKILLS

Appearing calm and collected is a public stance, but be sure to master the details. People feel more relaxed with someone whose demeanor radiates assurance and warmth.

What makes people uncomfortable? Restless hands, tapping toes, and squirming bodies. What makes people more comfortable? Good eye contact, poise, and genuine interest.

Being calm and collected is also important during an interview, whether for work, school, or a newspaper. Never answer questions immediately: wait a few seconds, compose your thoughts, and respond slowly and confidently.

Phase 3 | MAKING THE A-LIST

Phase 3 | MAKING THE A-LIST

MENU

Meal	Recipe	Yield	Calories	P. No.
Breakfast	Poached Eggs over Spinach	(1 serving)	246	154
Lunch	Carrot and Thyme Soup	(2 servings)	224	183
Snack	Dip 1 sliced orange bell pepper in dressing of 2 teaspoons olive oil, 1 teaspoon of chopped fresh herbs (such as dill and basil), and 1 tablespoon balsamic vinegar		111	
Dinner	Broiled Tuna with Tarragon Sauce	(1 serving)	264	157
	Brown Rice Pilaf	(1 serving)	134	180
Dessert	Thin Apple Tart	(1 serving)		205
	or 1 peach		61	
Total			1139	

EXERCISE

Let's use today to stretch out, walk, and recuperate from yesterday's double circuit. Even if you feel great, resist the temptation to overexert yourself. If your conscience bothers you, go for a very brisk walk in the park, around the block, or in any wide open space. Get rid of that nasty lactic acid, and get ready for tomorrow!

GROOMING TIP

When appoaching eye makeup, eye primer is a great place to start. Eye primer has a creamy consistency and neutralizes the color of the eyelid, as well as conceals any discoloration around the eye. Eye primer also helps eyeshadow colors to be more "true." It also wards off creasing. Your neutralizer should be beige or whitish in color—not the same color as foundation or concealer.

When buying eyeshadow, choose colors that work well together. Don't forget to pick out a highlighter. The highlighter should be a lighter color than the other colors, such as pale pink, champagne, or bone.

Tools are very important when applying eyeshadow. Throw out your sponge-tip applicators! I much prefer brushes, because they assist in even, accurate application.

Once you have all the right tools, application is easy! Begin by neutralizing your eyelid with the eye primer. Then, dip your brush into the eyeshadow, being sure to tap off the excess. Start applying from the inner corner of your eye, working to the outer corner, and finish by coloring in the lid. Add highlighter under the brow.

Don't forget mascara, which will help to bring out the shape of the eye. Black mascara is best, and will make eyes look bigger. If you don't want to go that dramatic, get as close to black as you can, with black/brown or deep green mascara.

Apply mascara slowly, beginning from the root. Wiggle the wand back and forth, then hold it firm to the lash and sweep the bristles up in one motion.

SELF-CONFIDENCE SKILLS

Remember the "talk show" entrance from a few days ago? Today you are going to rehearse a "first impression" that is more suitable for a business meeting or professional encounter.

Go back to the "waiting area" of the "television studio," well out of view of your mirror. This time, pretend that you are the Dalai Lama, Albert Schweitzer, or Mother Teresa accepting a humanitarian award. Walk gracefully toward the mirror, turn fully forward, and give a slight smile, nodding your head forward about an inch but still standing as tall as possible. Role-play this "entrance" about nine or ten times. It's much more dignified and respectful, an entrance well-suited for a meeting with your teacher, employer, guidance counselor, or even your parents.

Remind yourself each time: "I'm attending the Nobel Prize ceremony, the crowds are giving me a standing ovation, and the curtains are parting for my entrance."

Let your imagination shape the contours of your smile, the angle of your head, and the warmth of your eyes. Unlike that chorus girl in the musical "42nd Street," you are going out there as a star, and the physical "imprint" of assumed body language can eventually become a learned and thus permanent attribute.

Phase 3 | MAKING THE A-LIST

MENU

Meal	Recipe	Yield	Calories	P. No.
Breakfast	All-Bran with Apples and Cinnamon	(1 serving)	252	146
Lunch	Beet Salad	(1 serving)	278	190
Snack	Have $1/4$ cup whole-milk ricotta cheese mixed with 1 tablespoon apricot preserves and $1/4$ teaspoon pure almond extract; stir well to combine. Add 2 chopped fresh or canned (juice or water packed) apricots		140	TK
Dinner	Chicken au Citron	(1 serving)	245	167
	Zucchini and Bell Peppers with Pine Nuts	(1 serving)	117	176
Dessert	Winter Fruit Salad	(1 serving)	135	201
Total			1167	

EXERCISE

Back to business. Have you noticed how your posture has improved throughout the day? That's just one of the many benefits of our exercise circuits. Your friends, family, and colleagues will notice the others!

Exercise	Reps/Counts	Sets
Squats	12	3
Push-Ups	12	3
Back Row	12	3
Lunge	12 left leg / 12 right leg	3
Shoulder Press	12	3
One-Arm Row	12 with each arm	3
Plank	30 seconds, then 8 leg lifts on each side	3
Reverse Crunch	12	3

Do two circuits today!

FASHION TIP

Shoes are an important part of any outfit. Make sure you have at least one pair of black and brown shoes in appropriate styles. This goes for both men and women.

Shoe care requires a personal relationship with your local shoe-repair store, just as your wardrobe does with a dry cleaner—you will get better results if you show up and explain your wishes instead of relying on anonymous service.

Shoes last much longer if you polish them monthly, letting them dry at room temperature. For men's shoes, always use shoe blocks and store your shoes in cloth bags—then you are ready to travel with an extra pair that is already neat and clean.

INTERPERSONAL SKILLS

Coming in "first" is a winning attribute in the world of sports, beauty contests and politics. In social situations, however, you'll impress people even more if you're in "second place." Here's how and why it works.

Imagine you're on a date with a very special somebody. How can you show respect, deference, even protection, all at the same time? Just remember the words, "After you." When entering a movie theater, getting on the bus or even entering your own home, always let the other person go first. It's flattering, courteous and warm, all at the same time.

"After you" applies not just to opening a door, stepping aside, and letting someone else walk ahead. It's also a useful skill while engaging in conversations. Don't speak out immediately, but make sure that the other person has extra time to formulate thoughts and say what's on his or her mind. "What do you think?" typically wins more friends than "Listen to me."

Respect, deference, courtesy—"After you" represents the way you should live your life.

Phase 3 | MAKING THE A-LIST

MENU

Meal	Recipe	Yield	Calories	P. No.
Breakfast	Sweet Bell Pepper and Spinach Omelet	(1 serving)	224	152
Lunch	Mushroom and Barley Soup	(2 servings)	514	184
Snack	Mix 6 ounces low-fat plain yogurt with 2 teaspoons dried blueberries or raisins		125	
Dinner	Salmon a l'Orange	(1 serving)	368	159
Dessert	Acai and Berries Popsicles or watermelon– 1 cup diced	(1 serving)	76 46	202
Total			1307	

EXERCISE

Today, we'll take a break from the exercise circuits but not from exercise: if you are in an artistic mood—or the weather is bad—have your own private danceathon. While listening to your favorite up-tempo songs, indulge your fantasies, raise your heart rate, and enjoy your physicality. This isn't a chore or a homework assignment: it's fun. Of course, you might prefer a brisk walk—but why not a little self-indulgence that's good for you?

HAIR TIP

Making your hair look thicker can be accomplished in two different ways. First, select the appropriate hair products and develop a strict volumizing routine using a volumizing shampoo, conditioner, and volumizing spray.

Second, consider the use of hair extensions, which is actually the best way to achieve thickness, texture, and depth. For the best results, have your extensions put in by a professional. Also, find the right color and texture in order for the hair extensions to look as natural as possible.

SELF-CONFIDENCE SKILLS

The average American eats between 30 and 35 meals in an automobile each year. Most of these meals consist of high-calorie foods and beverages. Not only are Americans eating more food than ever, but they are eating it faster Your task today is to determine how you can limit eating "on the run," substituting leisurely "sit-down" lunches, suppers, and dinners for stress-filled "stand-up" or "motorized" meals.

If you have not already done so, you need to find a way to break this habit, and here is a suggestion. Plan a very special dinner date with a spouse, lover, or "significant other." Choose a restaurant where you can sit down and really enjoy the meal and each other's company. Take your time. Make your food choices wisely. Savor the meal, savor the conversation, and savor the companionship.

Making wise food choices should be a part of your daily routine by now. But judgment is especially important when you are with a spouse, lover, or close friend. You may be tempted to throw caution to the winds. Don't you dare. Special meals with special people deserve special food selection as well.

Phase 3 | MAKING THE A-LIST

MENU

Meal	Recipe	Yield	Calories	P. No.
Breakfast	Oatmeal with Raisins and Berries	(1 serving)	221	149
Lunch	Pasta with Vegetables and Sundried Tomatoes	(1 serving)	347	181
Snack	Pear and Almond Bruschetta	(1 serving)	94	199
Dinner	Chicken Cacciatora	(1 serving)	489	168
Dessert	Chocolate Square with Raspberry Coulis	(1 serving)	138	203
Total			1289	

EXERCISE

Today you're going to graduate to the triple superset, three full circuits of your exercise routine—now embedded into your muscle memory so carefully that the moves and transitions might be almost automatic. Breathing is not automatic, however, so remember to inhale and exhale deeply as you go.

Exercise	Reps/Counts	Sets
Squats	12	3
Push-Ups	12	3
Back Row	12	3
Lunge	12 left leg / 12 right leg	3
Shoulder Press	12	3
One-Arm Row	12 with each arm	3
Plank	30 seconds, then 8 leg lifts on each side	3
Reverse Crunch	12	3

Do three circuits today!

GROOMING TIP

Contouring helps to enhance the shape of one's face. It is a very fine art—sculpting is a better word—that helps to define the jawline, chin, and cheekbones.

I always start by using a soft shade of brown for contouring. The color should mimic the natural shadow between your chin and your neck. Note that these colors are usually taupe-y brown—not orange. Apply the contour color with a soft brush directly onto the area that concerns you, such as a fuller chin or neck area. The color will make the skin look more recessed, therefore resulting in a firmer, more sculptural appearance.

INTERPERSONAL SKILLS

Personal magnetism has something in common with the magnetism you learned about in high school physics: opposites attract. We are often captivated by and drawn to people who are quite different from us.

This phenomenon can produce unusually intimate and especially romantic relationships. However, there are inherent problems when two quite different individuals work, travel, or bond together, but fortunately these need not evolve into friction or animosity.

Be assured that you will never find anyone who shares all of your political, social, religious, cultural, and philosophical values. Finding lifelong companionship or an intimate friendship is an astounding achievement in itself. And longevity in relationships often requires a conscious effort at accommodation, compromise, and understanding.

Therefore try to defuse any negativity before it takes hold. You will never agree entirely with anyone else on the planet, so often it is best to be quiet, "agree to disagree," and concentrate on the blessings of friendship, companionship, and respect.

Phase 3 | MAKING THE A-LIST

MENU

Meal	Recipe	Yield	Calories	P. No.
Breakfast	Orange Wheat Muffin	(1 serving)	202	151
Lunch	Belgian Endive with Gorgonzola and Walnut	(2 servings)	396	191
Snack	Have 2 tablespoons sunflower seeds and 1 tablespoon dried blueberries or		127	
	$1/_2$ pink or red grapefruit		53	
Dinner	Broiled Salmon with Herbs de Provence	(1 serving)	316	160
	Brown Rice Pilaf	(1 serving)	134	180
Dessert	Have 1 sliced banana with 1 tablespoon chopped walnuts		154	
Total			1329	

EXERCISE

Time to stretch again; you'll find that you need this more frequently, rather than less, as you get stronger. Regeneration of muscle protein—not to mention its enlargement—depends on regular stretching, and walking is an ideal way to do it.

FASHION TIP

Treat your clothes as the invaluable possessions they are. Do not drop them on the floor. Doing so equals abusing them. Always fold knits and put them away immediately after you take them off. Hang up any piece that belongs in the closet as well.

Remember that finding a good dry cleaner is crucial to looking stylish and well turned out. Many fashion experts have a wrinkle fetish and consider pressing garments mandatory, but reliable cleaners can also help remove stains as well as change buttons and do alterations.

Make sure you have proper hangers, not the wire ones from the cleaners. Over time, wire will ruin the shape of your clothes. Men: hang your pants properly so that the hanger does not accidentally crease the cuffs.

SELF-CONFIDENCE SKILLS

Today's exercise is to take a close look at yourself, where you feel quite confident, whether it be personal appearance, academics, athletics, business, social relationships, or something else. Now note the areas where you don't feel as confident. Monitor your feelings and "self-talk." Resist such statements as:

"I will never have as many friends as my neighbor does, so why should I keep the weight off?"

"When I go to the health club, I swim more slowly than anyone else, so this diet is not working for me."

"Someone else got that promotion at work, so I really need a food binge to cheer me up."

Notice that these unrealistic personal myths are based on comparisons. They falsely imply that people are failures if they do not have love and approval from every significant person in their life, that they must be thoroughly competent in everything they do, or that they must always gain recognition and praise for their achievements.

Nobody is perfect. You have heard this before, but do you really believe it? Can you accept yourself the way you are with all your strengths and weaknesses? If so, you will engage in the realistic, rational, positive, optimistic kind of "self-talk" that will keep off those pounds you have worked so hard to shed.

Please give yourself credit for everything that you do well. Please refrain from criticizing yourself whenever you goof up. Please approach new experiences as opportunities to learn rather than contests to win or lose. Whenever a negative thought or feeling pops up, replace it with something that is upbeat. Then you will have the emotional intelligence and the self-confidence to stick to what *The Park Avenue Diet* has taught you.

Phase 3 | MAKING THE A-LIST

MENU

Meal	Recipe	Yield	Calories	P. No.
Breakfast	Poached Eggs over Spinach	(1 serving)	246	154
Lunch	Spinach and Onion Soup	(2 servings)	394	185
Snack	Have $1/2$ cup red grapes with 1 tablespoon walnuts or 1 plum		104

30 | |
Dinner	Turkey Breast with Sage	(1 serving)	341	171
	Zucchini and Bell Peppers with Pine Nuts	(1 serving)	117	176
Dessert	Thin Apple Tart	(1 serving)	160	205
Total			1362	

EXERCISE

Three circuits of our exercise routine will enliven our final week together. Have you noticed how your breathing and posture have improved? Have other people noticed anything? What a compliment it is when your friends recognize the results you've achieved, particularly when it concerns bodily physique. But let's get back to the matters at hand—your triple superset.

Exercise	Reps/Counts	Sets
Squats	12	3
Push-Ups	12	3
Back Row	12	3
Lunge	12 left leg / 12 right leg	3
Shoulder Press	12	3
One-Arm Row	12 with each arm	3
Plank	30 seconds, then 8 leg lifts on each side	3
Reverse Crunch	12	3

Do three circuits today!

HAIR TIP

If you are concerned about the effect of steam rooms on your hair, fear not. Steam rooms are great for one's hair. They're a perfect place to apply a conditioning treatment because the conditioner adheres better to your hair when the air is so full of moisture.

The best salons actually have streamers for conditioning treatments because the heat and moisture make for really healthy-looking hair.

INTERPERSONAL SKILLS

What do we call people who think that "flattery will get you nowhere"? Lonely. Almost everyone likes to be noticed and made to feel special.

Giving a compliment to someone else is also a reflection of your own self-confidence. Be sincere, never obsequious, and use flattery with restraint.

Your body language and eye contact can also radiate your sincerity; if you are giving false praise, it will be apparent in the tone of your voice, facial expressions, or lack of comfort.

Don't give a compliment for the sole purpose of getting something in return. Give a compliment because you know that the praise will make someone feel good and that it is deserved.

Phase 3 | MAKING THE A-LIST

Phase 3 | MAKING THE A-LIST

MENU

Meal	Recipe	Yield	Calories	P. No.
Breakfast	Homemade Granola with Pumpkin Yogurt	(1 serving)	313	148
Lunch	Macaroni and Cheese a la Francaise	(2 servings)	340	182
Snack	Zucchini Stuffed with Tuna	(2 servings)	188	200
Dinner	Trout with Horseradish	(1 serving)	263	161
	Green Beans with Mushroom	(1 serving)	94	179
Dessert	Winter Fruit Salad	(1 serving)	135	
Total			1333	

EXERCISE

We're nearing the end of our time together as part of *The Park Avenue Diet*. Today we're doing a triple superset, just like yesterday. Be careful about your breathing patterns, and always keep your form excellent, counting slowly to achieve maximal results.

Exercise	Reps/Counts	Sets
Squats	12	3
Push-Ups	12	3
Back Row	12	3
Lunge	12 left leg / 12 right leg	?
Shoulder Press	12	3
One-Arm Row	12 with each arm	3
Plank	30 seconds, then 8 leg lifts on each side	3
Reverse Crunch	12	3

Do three circuits today!

GROOMING TIP

Most of us have at least one blemish that we need to conceal. If so, follow the steps below.

What you should always do first is apply foundation. This way, you start with seeing how much coverage you can get—for some people, this first step might be enough to conceal the blemish.

If not, apply a concealer on top of the foundation. The color of the concealer should match the foundation, and the consistency of the concealer should be creamy in texture but not greasy. Use a pointed, stiff brush for precise placement of the concealer to really target the blemish. Then use a fan brush, not a dense brush, to apply a light dusting of translucent loose powder over your entire face. This will help set your makeup.

SELF-CONFIDENCE SKILLS

Learning theory goes back to the Greek philosopher Aristotle. He recognized that enjoyment was the result of some positive achievement. Today's psychologists would call this one's "personal best" or "peak performance."

The Park Avenue Diet has taught you several ways to excel. And now that you feel better about yourself socially, physically, and spiritually, you don't need to use food as a "comfort blanket." You have transformed your thoughts, feelings, and behaviors for the better. Review these exercises from time to time.

There is more to life than losing weight. And now you can move on to discover what that may be for you. Good luck!

Phase 3 | MAKING THE A-LIST

MENU

Meal	Recipe	Yield	Calories	P. No.
Breakfast	Sweet Bell Pepper and Spinach Omelet	(1 serving)	224	152
Lunch	Chicken Salad with Fruit	(1 serving)	376	194
Snack	Dip 7 cherry tomatoes in 1 tablespoon olive tapenade or 1 peach		97 61	
Dinner	Tuscan Beef Stew	(1 serving)	434	172
Dessert	Chocolate Square with Raspberry Coulis	(1 serving)	138	203
Total			1269	

EXERCISE

One last opportunity to focus on stretching before the final push—so take a walk, ride a bicycle, or swim, and compliment yourself on a job well done, where you are the principle beneficiary.

FASHION TIP

By now, you know how to put together a properly fitting and elegantly coordinated outfit for any occasion. Show off your newfound expertise by choosing a special item of clothing that will make you feel like the confident person you are!

Are you planning for an intimate evening with a special friend? In order to look your best, have your most spectacular outfit cleaned, pressed, and ready to dazzle—that way, you can relax and enjoy yourself even more.

INTERPERSONAL SKILLS

When you leave your house or apartment, be sure that you look presentable. You never know whom you might meet, so prepare your outfit, hair, skin, and breath accordingly. This "social skill" should be done before you interact with anyone: a trip to the store, the mailbox, or the mall may start out alone, but surprises do happen, especially pleasant ones.

Phase 3 | MAKING THE A-LIST

MENU

Meal	Recipe	Yield	Calories	P. No.
Breakfast	All-Bran with Apples and Cinnamon	(1 serving)	252	146
Lunch	Pumpkin Soup and Pepitas	(2 servings)	356	186
Snack	Have 1/4 cup whole-milk ricotta cheese mixed with 1 tablespoon apricot preserves and 1/4 teaspoon pure almond extract; stir well to combine. Add 2 chopped fresh or canned (juice or water packed) apricots		140	
Dinner	Sea Bass with Mango Coulis	(1 serving)	329	162
	Brown Rice Pilaf	(1 serving)	134	180
Dessert	Have 1 sliced banana with 1 tablespoon chopped walnuts		154	
Total			1365	

EXERCISE

Have you mastered the three-circuit exercise routine yet? Don't feel bad if it's still a "work-in-progress." It may take you a few days or weeks to become truly comfortable with this challenging but time-efficient program. Be sure to include rest/stretching days as we've done in weeks past. Whenever you need a reminder or want to double-check if you're doing everything correctly, don't hesitate to read back through the entire exercise section. Congratulations—and enjoy the results!

Exercise	Reps/Counts	Sets
Squats	12	3
Push-Ups	12	3
Back Row	12	3
Lunge	12 left leg / 12 right leg	3
Shoulder Press	12	3

One-Arm Row	12 with each arm	3
Plank	30 seconds, then 8 leg lifts on each side	3
Reverse Crunch	12	3

Do three circuits today!

HAIR TIP

Experts are always asked how to make hair more healthy and shiny. There are two tasks you can perform to get optimal health and shine back into your hair. First, your hair lacks shine because the cuticle of the hair is open. This in effect prevents light from reflecting off your hair, making it look dull. The proper hair products will help and close the cuticle, allowing light to reflect and giving your hair a shiny appearance.

A glaze is a treatment that is used to create a shine or enhance your hair color whether it is colored or natural. How will this look on you? Ask your stylist.

SELF-CONFIDENCE SKILLS

In addition to intellectual intelligence and emotional intelligence, many psychologists have suggested that it is important to develop spiritual intelligence. Your spiritual intelligence will provide insights that will help you to take what you have learned by working with *The Park Avenue Diet* and spread the good news around. Happiness and joy are much more fun if they are shared. And you now have the self-confidence to spread the good news.

Self-confidence can help you teach friends and family members how to identify their negative personal myths. You can boost their self-confidence by giving compliments and praise when it is appropriate. This will reinforce their positive thoughts, feelings, and behavior. At the same time, you can lend a helping hand when someone is in need, even if the needy person is not a member of your extended family or your circle of friends. Loving your neighbor as yourself is at the core of the world's great religions, and you can make a difference in someone else's life every day. Providing compassion and love in the right amount at an appropriate time is the true mark of spiritual intelligence.

When you decided to lose weight, you probably never thought you would also lose negative personal myths, negative attitudes, negative feelings, and negative behaviors. But if you can lose one piece of this cumbersome emotional baggage, you are on your way to losing the rest of these unnecessary burdens. Good riddance. Without them, you can really fly!

Phase 3 | MAKING THE A-LIST

MENU

Meal	Recipe	Yield	Calories	P. No.
Breakfast	Muesli with Peach and Almond	(1 serving)	211	147
Lunch	Four Bean Salad	(2 servings)	490	193
Snack	Mix 6 ounces low-fat plain yogurt with 2 teaspoons dried blueberries or raisins		125	
Dinner	Turkey Breast with Sage	(1 serving)	341	171
	Zucchini and Bell Peppers with Pine Nuts	(1 serving)	117	176
Dessert	Winter Fruit Salad	(1 serving)	135	201
Total			1419	

EXERCISE

The triple superset is your goal. You'll want to master it so you can do it comfortably 3 to 4 times per week. After you've finished today, pause to reflect on the benefits of exercise: you've proven yourself capable of reinventing your muscle structure, shrinking fat cells and growing sexy lean muscle, while aligning and lengthening your spinal column.

This will, in turn, inspire you to other challenges, whether they are personal, professional, academic, or social. You'll feel different about yourself as you get stronger, and this will be apparent to everyone around you. Enjoy the results of your hard work!

Exercise	Reps/Counts	Sets
Squats	12	3
Push-Ups	12	3
Back Row	12	3
Lunge	12 left leg / 12 right leg	3
Shoulder Press	12	3
One-Arm Row	12 with each arm	3
Plank	30 seconds, then 8 leg lifts on each side	3
Reverse Crunch	12	3

Do three circuits today!

Well done! You're pulled and pressed to be your best—now go enjoy the fabulous results!

GROOMING TIP

It is extremely important to know when you have too much makeup on. Many women feel they have to cover their flaws and therefore they tend to wear too much.

If your makeup smudges easily, you are probably wearing way too much. Proper makeup application looks fresh for hours, whereas heavy makeup smears easily and tends not to last. To determine if you are wearing too much makeup, look at yourself in a mirror near a window or other source of natural light (or, you can even take a mirror and step outside to look at yourself). If it looks to *you* like you are wearing too much makeup, you will look that way to others, too.

INTERPERSONAL SKILLS

At last it's time for you to put your interpersonal skills to use. There are many new people for you to meet and wonderful new paths to follow on your life journey—but don't do it alone.

Have you always dreamed of meeting that special someone? Longed for an intimate relationship but have been too shy to consider it? Since you've developed a positive sense of self, you'll find it surprisingly easy to make friends, even to find a significant other and forge a bond that will enrich both your lives.

No need to be lonely or to turn inward unnecessarily. You can meet someone special and make your life happier. Perhaps you were previously too insecure to speak to someone you admired at school, at work, at the mall, or at a club. Maybe you didn't know what to say and stared at the floor while your body language sent out a "stay-away" message. Those days are gone forever.

The self-confidence you have developed will help you radiate poise and start a conversation. Give a glance, smile, and speak up. Go ahead, you are worth knowing.

You've learned to like yourself. Now it's time for someone else to like you.

Phase 4 | MAKING THE A-LIST

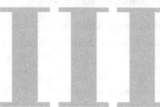

THE PARK AVENUE
RECIPES

What follows here are the original recipes from Chef Marie for the menus listed in the Six-Week Park Avenue Diet. The recipes are intended to be simple to make, and use readily available ingredients. If you'd like to experiment with them, by all means do so. Enjoy the process *and* the results!

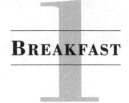

BREAKFAST

All-Bran with Apples and Cinnamon

1 cup all bran flakes

1/2 cup low-fat milk

1/4 cup apples

1 tablespoon raisins

1 teaspoon flaxseeds

Cinnamon to taste

1. In a bowl mix the cereal with the milk. Top with the apples, raisins, and flaxseeds. Sprinkle cinnamon and serve immediately.

YIELD 1 SERVING:

252 Cal (14% from Fat, 13% from Protein, 73% from Carb);
9 g Protein; 5 g Tot Fat; 2 g Sat Fat; 1 g Mono Fat; 52 g Carb; 9 g Fiber; 23 g Sugar; 192 mg Calcium; 12 mg Iron; 345 mg Sodium; 10 mg Cholesterol (2% milk)

Muesli with Peach and Almond

1/2 cup muesli cereal

1/2 cup low-fat yogurt

2 teaspoons almonds, slivered or sliced

2 ounces peaches

Milk (optional)

1. In a bowl mix the cereal with the yogurt. If too thick, add a little milk to thin out. Top with the peaches, and almonds, and serve immediately.

YIELD 1 SERVING:

211 Cal (29% from Fat, 27% from Protein, 44% from Carb);
5 g Protein; 7 g Tot Fat; 3 g Sat Fat; 3 g Mono Fat; 24 g Carb; 2 g Fiber; 22 g Sugar; 467 mg Calcium; 1 mg Iron; 172 mg Sodium; 15 mg Cholesterol

Homemade Granola
with Pumpkin Yogurt

1/4 cup honey

1/4 cup vegetable oil

2 teaspoons pumpkin pie spices

1 teaspoon almond extract

1/2 teaspoon orange extract

3 1/2 cups old fashioned oats, uncooked

1/4 cup sliced almonds

1/4 cup chopped walnuts

5 cups plain low-fat yogurt (ten 1/2 cups of low-fat yogurt)

10 tablespoons canned pumpkin puree

Milk (optional)

1. Preheat the oven to 350°F.
2. In a bowl, mix the honey, spices, oil, and extracts. Stir in the oats and nuts.
3. Mix well and spread over a greased cookie sheet.
4. Bake for 10 minutes. Stir and continue to bake for another 10 minutes or until golden brown. Cool completely and break apart.
5. Mix the pumpkin puree with the yogurt. If too thick, add a little milk to thin out. Blend the mixture with the prepared granola and serve immediately.

YIELD: 10 SERVINGS

313 Cal (36% from Fat, 15% from Protein, 49% from Carb); 12 g Protein; 13 g Tot Fat; 3 g Sat Fat; 4 g Mono Fat; 39 g Carb; 4 g Fiber; 19 g Sugar; 259 mg Calcium; 2 mg Iron; 89 mg Sodium; 7 mg Cholesterol (1serving = 1/2 cup granola, 1/2 cup low-fat yogurt, and 1 tablespoon pumpkin puree)

Oatmeal with Raisins and Berries

1/2 cup oatmeal

1 cup hot water or milk (regular or 2%)

2 teaspoons walnuts

1 teaspoon raisins

2 ounces berries

1 teaspoon flaxseeds

1. Place the oatmeal in a bowl, add the hot liquid, and mix well.
2. Mix in the walnuts, raisins, and flaxseeds. Top with the berries and serve immediately.

YIELD: 1 SERVING (WITH WATER)

221 Cal (21% from Fat, 11% from Protein, 68% from Carb);
7 g Protein; 6 g Tot Fat; 1 g Sat Fat; 1 g Mono Fat; 41 g Carb; 10 g Fiber; 5 g Sugar; 45 mg Calcium; 2 mg Iron; 8 mg Sodium; 0 mg Cholesterol

---

YIELD: 1 SERVING (WITH 2% MILK)

343 Cal (26% from Fat, 16% from Protein, 58% from Carb);
15 g Protein; 11 g Tot Fat; 4 g Sat Fat; 2 g Mono Fat; 52 g Carb; 10 g Fiber; 17 g Sugar; 326 mg Calcium; 2 mg Iron; 103 mg Sodium; 20 mg Cholesterol

Buckwheat Crêpes with Salmon

1/2 cup all-purpose flour

1/2 cup buckwheat flour

2 eggs

1 tablespoon honey

2 tablespoons vegetable oil

1 cup milk

1 teaspoon vanilla extract

Vegetable oil for greasing the pan

Pinch Salt

10 tablespoons crème fraiche

10 smoked salmon slices (about 10 ounces)

Fresh dill, minced

1 lemon

1. Place the flour in a bowl. Blend in the eggs, oil, honey, vanilla, and salt. Slowly whisk in the milk. Strain and let the batter rest for 30 minutes in the refrigerator. Before use, add a little water to thin it out.
2. Heat a nonstick pan or crêpe pan over medium heat. Soak a small piece of paper towel with 1 teaspoon oil and wipe the greased towel quickly over the pan. Add enough batter and swirl to cover the entire bottom. Cook until golden brown and turn over. Cook until golden brown. Repeat this process until all the crêpe batter is used.
3. Spread each crêpe with 1 tablespoon of crème fraiche and sprinkle dill. Top with a smoked salmon slice and sprinkle lemon juice. Fold or roll the crêpe and serve immediately.

Crème fraiche may be replaced with sour cream.

YIELD: 10 SERVINGS

181 Cal (51% from Fat, 21% from Protein, 28% from Carb);
9 g Protein; 10 g Tot Fat; 4 g Sat Fat; 3 g Mono Fat; 13 g Carb; 1 g Fiber; 3 g Sugar; 53 mg Calcium; 1 mg Iron; 255 mg Sodium; 71 mg Cholesterol

Orange Wheat Muffin

1 cup unbleached all-purpose
    flour

1/2 cup whole wheat flour

1/2 cup flaxseed meal

1/3 cup honey

1 teaspoon baking soda

1 tablespoon baking powder

1/4 teaspoon salt

1 teaspoon orange extract

1 teaspoon orange zest

2 large eggs

2 tablespoons canola oil

1/2 cup pumpkin puree (can)

1 cup low-fat yogurt

12 tablespoons orange
    marmalade

1. Preheat the oven to 375° F.
2. Blend the flours, flaxseed meal, honey, baking soda, baking powder, and salt in a mixing bowl. Blend in the orange extract, orange zest, canola oil, eggs, pumpkin puree, and yogurt, and mix until well incorporated.
3. Fill muffin pan and bake for 25 minutes or until cooked through and golden brown.
4. Serve each muffin with 1 tablespoon of orange marmalade.

 ▶ *You may replace 2 eggs with 4 egg whites.*
 ▶ *Careful, this recipe can act like a laxative.*

YIELD: 12 SERVINGS

181 Cal (51% from Fat, 21% from Protein, 28% from Carb);
5 g Protein; 4 g Tot Fat; 1 g Sat Fat; 2 g Mono Fat; 39 g Carb; 2 g Fiber; 22 g Sugar; 126 mg Calcium; 1 mg Iron; 317 mg Sodium; 42 mg Cholesterol (1 muffin and 1 tablespoon orange marmalade)

Sweet Bell Pepper and Spinach Omelet

8 eggs

1 tablespoon milk

2 teaspoons olive oil

2 ounces onions, diced (about 1/2 small onion)

2 garlic cloves, minced

10 ounces bell peppers; seeded and sliced (one yellow and one red, medium size)

8 ounces cooked spinach, chopped

2 tablespoons fresh salad herbs, minced

Salt and pepper to taste

1. Heat the oil in a nonstick pan over medium heat.
2. Add the onions and sauté until translucent.
3. Add the garlic, and bell peppers, and cook for 2 to 3 minutes. Season to taste and spread the vegetables evenly over the bottom of the pan.
4. In a bowl, beat the eggs, milk, and season to taste. Add the egg mixture to the vegetables and let the eggs slightly set.
5. Spread the spinach, reduce heat, and continue to cook for 2 to 3 minutes. Fold in half, cook for another minute, and serve immediately.

YIELD: 4 SERVINGS

224 Cal (56% from Fat, 30% from Protein, 14% from Carb);
17 g Protein; 14 g Tot Fat; 4 g Sat Fat; 6 g Mono Fat; 8 g Carb; 3 g Fiber; 4 g Sugar; 118 mg Calcium; 4 mg Iron; 200 mg Sodium; 491 mg Cholesterol

Country Frittata

8 eggs

2 tablespoons milk

2 teaspoons olive oil

2 green onions, chopped

2 garlic cloves, minced

8 ounces zucchini, sliced (about 1 large zucchini)

4 ounces red bell pepper, sliced (about 1 medium bell pepper)

2 tablespoons shredded Parmesan or Romano

2 tablespoons fresh salad herbs, minced

Salt and pepper to taste

1. Heat the oil in a nonstick pan over medium heat.
2. Add the garlic, and zucchini, and sauté for 2 to 3 minutes.
3. Add the bell pepper, green onions, herbs, and continue to sauté for 2 minutes. Spread the vegetables evenly over the bottom of the pan.
4. In a bowl, beat the eggs, milk, cheese, and season to taste. Add the egg mixture to the vegetables and let the eggs set.
5. Reduce heat and continue to cook for 2 to 3 minutes. Flip over and continue to cook until golden brown. Transfer to a platter, cut in wedges, and serve immediately.

YIELD: 4 SERVINGS

Per Serving: 230 Cal (59% from Fat, 30% from Protein, 11% from Carb); 17 g Protein; 15 g Tot Fat; 5 g Sat Fat; 6 g Mono Fat; 6 g Carb; 1 g Fiber; 4 g Sugar; 127 mg Calcium; 3 mg Iron; 223 mg Sodium; 494 mg Cholesterol

Poached Eggs over Spinach

8 eggs

4 teaspoons olive oil

6 cups fresh baby spinach leaves

4 tablespoons cream, hot (optional)

Four pinches nutmeg

Four pinches paprika

Salt and pepper to taste

1. Grease 4 small casserole dishes with olive oil and set aside.
2. Fill a large pan with water and bring to a boil over high heat.
3. Meanwhile, preheat a steamer. Place the spinach into the steamer basket and cook until barely wilted.
4. Reduce the heat under the boiling water to a point where the water barely bubbles. Break the eggs and slide them one by one into the simmering water. Make sure the eggs do not touch. Cook until the whites are set and firm to the touch (about 3 minutes).
5. Divide the spinach equally among the casseroles. Spread one tablespoon of cream per casserole. Sprinkle nutmeg and season to taste.
6. Using a slotted spoon carefully remove each egg. Place two eggs on top of the prepared casserole. Sprinkle with paprika and serve immediately.

YIELD: 4 SERVINGS

Per Serving: 246 Cal (69% from Fat, 26% from Protein, 4% from Carb);
16 g Protein; 19 g Tot Fat; 6 g Sat Fat; 9 g Mono Fat; 3 g Carb; 1 g Fiber; 1 g Sugar; 111 mg Calcium; 3 mg Iron; 201 mg Sodium; 501 mg Cholesterol

FISH AND SEAFOOD

Tuna Provençal

1 tablespoon olive oil

Four 5-ounce tuna steaks

2 pounds tomatoes

8 ounces onions, sliced

8 ounces green bell peppers;
seeded, ribs removed, and
sliced

Salt and pepper to taste

8 ounces yellow bell peppers;
seeded, ribs removed, and
sliced

2 tablespoons garlic cloves,
minced

2 pinches herbs de Provence

1 bunch fresh basil, shredded

1/2 cup brown rice

1. Make a small X incision on the top and bottom of each tomatoe. Blanch the tomatoes for 20 seconds. Remove and place in ice-cold water to stop the cooking process. Peel, seed, and slice the tomatoes.
2. Cook the rice according to package instructions.
3. Heat the oil in a large pan over high heat. Add the tuna and brown. Turn over and cook for 2 minutes. Remove the fish and set aside on a plate.
4. Deglaze the pan with a little water. To deglaze, add a liquid (such as wine, stock, or water) and swirl to dissolve cooked particles on the bottom and side of the pan.
5. Add the onions and cook for 2 minutes.
6. Add the garlic, tomatoes, bell peppers, herbs de Provence, and sauté for 2 minutes.
7. Slide in the fish, cover, and cook for 20 minutes over low heat. Remove the fillets and set aside in a platter. Cover with aluminum foil to keep warm. Mix the basil into the vegetables and season to taste. Pour over the fish and serve immediately with the rice.

▶ *The fish and rice may be refrigerated separately up to 2 days.*

▶ *The fish and rice may be frozen separately up to 1 month.*

YIELD: 4 SERVINGS

328 Cal (19% from Fat, 31% from Protein, 50% from Carb);
26 g Protein; 7 g Tot Fat; 1 g Sat Fat; 3 g Mono Fat; 42 g Carb; 6 g Fiber; 4 g Sugar; 60 mg
Calcium; 2 mg Iron; 53 mg Sodium; 35 mg Cholesterol

Broiled Tuna
with Tarragon Sauce

1 tablespoon olive oil

Four 5-ounce tuna fillets

1 small shallot, minced

1 garlic clove, minced

1/2 cup white wine (Sauvignon Blanc)

Salt and pepper to taste

3/4 cup vegetable stock

2 tablespoons Dijon mustard

Cornstarch

2 tablespoons cream (optional)

8 fresh tarragon branches

Oil spray

1. Preheat the broiler.
2. Mince four tarragon branches and set aside. Heat the oil in a pan over high heat.
3. Add the shallot and garlic, and sauté for a minute. Add the wine, stock, and half the minced tarragon, and boil for 3 minutes. Strain and return liquid to the pan.
4. Add the mustard and mix briefly. Thicken with a little cornstarch mixed with water. Remove from heat and set aside.
5. Place the fillets on a greased cookie sheet. Rub the remaining tarragon branches on both sides of the fillets. Spray a little oil over the fillets.
6. Broil for 4 to 5 minutes. Turn over and spray a little more oil. Continue to broil until the flesh starts to flake. Remove the fillets and keep warm in a plate covered with aluminum foil.
7. Reheat the prepared sauce, add the cream and remaining minced tarragon, and bring to a boil. Adjust seasonings, pour over the fillets, and serve immediately.

Serve with Brown Rice Pilaf.

▶ *The fish and rice may be refrigerated separately up to 2 days.*
▶ *The fish and rice may be frozen separately up to 1 month.*

▶ *The amount of cornstarch and water mixture may vary depending on the amount of water rendered by the fish and the reduction process. To obtain the right thickness for a sauce: Dip a spoon in the sauce, turn it over, and make a line across with your finger. Tilt the spoon. If the sauce does not run over the line, it is the perfect thickness. If it does, you need to thicken with a little cornstarch and water mixture. After adding the mixture, you will need to bring the sauce to a boil. If it gets too thick, just add a little stock to thin out.*

YIELD: 4 SERVINGS

264 Cal (42% from Fat, 50% from Protein, 8% from Carb);
30 g Protein; 11 g Tot Fat; 3 g Sat Fat; 5 g Mono Fat; 5 g Carb; 0 g Fiber; 0 g Sugar; 45 mg Calcium; 2 mg Iron; 365 mg Sodium; 60 mg Cholesterol (cream)

Salmon à l'Orange

FOR THE FISH:

1 tablespoon olive oil

Four 5-ounce salmon fillets

1 shallot, sliced

2 oranges

1/4 cup orange juice, hot

1 teaspoon coriander seeds, crushed

1 teaspoon ground ginger

2 tablespoons fresh parsley, chopped

Salt and pepper to taste

FOR THE VEGETABLES:

1 pound carrots

1 pound broccoli

Salt and pepper to taste

For the fish:
1. With a zester remove the orange zests. Julienne the zests and set aside. Remove the white part of the oranges and separate the orange segments.
2. Grease an ovenproof pan just large enough to contain the fillets.
3. Add the fillets and sprinkle ginger, half the orange zest, a little salt, and pepper. Spread the shallots, orange segments, and parsley over the fillets.
4. Mix the hot orange juice with the coriander seeds and the remaining zests, and pour around the fillets. Cover with aluminum foil and bake for 15 to 20 minutes or until the fillets start to flake.
5. Remove from the oven and serve immediately with the steamed vegetables.

For the vegetables:
1. Preheat a steamer. Add the carrots and cook covered until you reach almost the desired tenderness.
2. Add the broccoli and continue to cook for 1 to 2 minutes. Transfer to a serving plate and season to taste.

▶ *The fish and vegetables may be refrigerated separately up to 2 days.*
▶ *The fish and vegetables may be frozen separately up to 1 month.*

YIELD: 4 SERVINGS

368 Cal (29% from Fat, 38% from Protein, 33% from Carb);
36 g Protein; 12 g Tot Fat; 3 g Sat Fat; 5 g Mono Fat; 31 g Carb; 9 g Fiber; 17 g Sugar; 488 mg Calcium; 3 mg Iron; 224 mg Sodium; 55 mg Cholesterol

Broiled Salmon with Herbs de Provence

FOR THE FISH:

2 tablespoons olive oil

Four 5-ounce salmon fillets

6 large pinches of herbs de Provence

1 lemon

Salt and pepper to taste

FOR THE VEGETABLES:

32 asparagus, trimmed (about 2 pounds of asparagus)

1 lemon, quartered

For the fish:
1. Preheat the broiler.
2. Place the fillets on a greased pan. Brush olive oil and sprinkle lemon juice over the fillets. Season with pepper and herbs de Provence.
3. Broil for 3 to 4 minutes. Turn over, brush with oil, and continue to broil for 3 to 4 minutes or until the salmon flesh start to flake.
4. Transfer to a serving platter, sprinkle lemon juice over the fillets and season with salt. Serve immediately with the prepared vegetables and lemon wedges.

For the vegetables:
1. Preheat a steamer. Place the asparagus in the steamer basket. Steam until desired tenderness.

▶ *The fish and vegetables may be refrigerated separately up to 2 days.*
▶ *The fish and vegetables may be frozen separately up to 1 month.*

YIELD: 4 SERVINGS

316 Cal (40% from Fat, 43% from Protein, 17% from Carb);
36 g Protein; 15 g Tot Fat; 3 g Sat Fat; 8 g Mono Fat; 15 g Carb; 7 g Fiber; 4 g Sugar; 440 mg Calcium; 6 mg Iron; 113 mg Sodium; 55 mg Cholesterol

Trout with Horseradish

1 tablespoon olive oil

Four 5-ounce trout, whole

3 tablespoons fresh parsley, minced

4 tablespoons prepared horseradish sauce (store bought)

Salt and pepper to taste

1. Preheat the broiler.
2. Clean the fish and pat dry. Sprinkle the inside of the trout with a little salt, pepper, oil, and parsley.
3. Place the trout on a greased baking pan. Rub a little olive oil over the trout skin.
4. Broil for 3 to 4 minutes.
5. Carefully turn over, brush with oil, and continue to broil for another 3 to 4 minutes. Serve immediately with the prepared horseradish sauce.

This recipe goes well with Green Beans with Mushrooms.

▸ *The fish and vegetables may be refrigerated separately up to 2 days.*
▸ *Not recommended for freezing.*

YIELD: 4 SERVINGS

263 Cal (48% from Fat, 45% from Protein, 7% from Carb);
30 g Protein; 14 g Tot Fat; 2 g Sat Fat; 8 g Mono Fat; 5 g Carb; 2 g Fiber; 1 g Sugar; 90 mg Calcium; 3 mg Iron; 123 mg Sodium; 82 mg Cholesterol

Sea Bass with Mango Coulis

FOR THE FISH:

1 tablespoon canola oil

Four 5-ounce sea bass fillets

2 mangos

1 jalapeno, seeded

2 tablespoons fresh cilantro, chopped

2 green onions, chopped

2 limes, juiced

1/4 cup low-fat yogurt

FOR THE VEGETABLES:

2 teaspoons olive oil

4 ounces red onions, sliced (about 1 small red onion)

2 red bell peppers; seeded, ribs removed, and sliced

1 yellow bell pepper, seeded, ribs removed, and sliced

1 tablespoon fresh cilantro

Salt and pepper to taste

For the fish:
1. In a blender puree the mango, jalapeno, cilantro, green onions, and 2 tablespoons lime juice. Transfer to a serving bowl and blend in the yogurt. Season to taste and refrigerate for later use.
2. Sprinkle the fish with a little pepper. Heat the oil in a nonstick pan over medium heat. Add the fillets pepper side down and brown. Turn over and cook for 2 minutes.
3. Add some lime juice and continue to cook until the flesh starts to flake.

For the vegetables:
1. Heat the oil in a pan over high heat. Add the onion and sauté quickly.
2. Add the bell peppers and cook for 3 minutes, mixing occasionally.
3. Mix in the cilantro and season to taste.
4. Serve the vegetables with the cooked fish and mango coulis.

▸ *The fish and vegetables may be refrigerated separately up to 2 days.*
▸ *The fish and vegetables may be frozen separately up to 1 month.*

YIELD: 4 SERVINGS

329 Cal (26% from Fat, 35% from Protein, 39% from Carb);
29 g Protein; 10 g Tot Fat; 2 g Sat Fat; 4 g Mono Fat; 32 g Carb; 4 g Fiber; 22 g Sugar; 71 mg Calcium; 1 mg Iron; 112 mg Sodium; 60 mg Cholesterol

Codfish with Ratatouille

2 tablespoons olive oil

Four 5-ounce cod fillets

1/2 pound zucchini, diced (about 2 medium zucchini)

1/2 pound eggplant, peeled and diced (about 1 medium eggplant)

1/2 pound onions, thinly sliced (about 1 large onion)

6 ounces red bell peppers, thinly sliced (about 1 large red bell pepper)

6 ounces yellow bell peppers, thinly sliced (about 1 large yellow bell pepper)

1 tablespoon garlic cloves, minced

1 pound tomatoes (about 3 large tomatoes)

3 tablespoons fresh parsley, minced

5 fresh basil leaves, minced

1 bay leaf

1/2 teaspoon herbs de Provence

Salt and pepper to taste

1. Make a small X incision into the tops and bottoms of the tomatoes. Heat some water over high heat and bring to a boil. Blanch the tomatoes for 20 seconds. Strain and immediately place the tomatoes in ice cold water to stop the cooking process. Peel, seed, and dice the tomatoes.
2. Heat 1 tablespoon of oil in a deep pan over medium heat. Add the onions and sauté until translucent. Add the zucchini, eggplant, bell peppers, garlic, tomatoes, herbs de Provence and bay leaf, and bring to a boil. Reduce heat, cover, and cook for 20 minutes.
3. Sprinkle the fish with a little pepper. Heat 1 tablespoon oil in a skillet and brown the fish on both sides. Slide the fillets into the ratatouille and continue to cook for 15 minutes (if the ratatouille is very liquid, leave uncovered; if not, cover.) Remove fillets and place on a serving platter. Cover with aluminum foil to keep warm. If the ratatouille is still too liquid, reduce uncovered over medium heat until it has the consistency of a sauce.
4. Add the parsley, and basil, and adjust seasonings to the ratatouille. Transfer to a serving bowl and serve immediately with the fillets.

> ► *The fish and vegetables may be refrigerated separately up to 2 days.*
> ► *The fish and vegetables may be frozen separately up to 1 month.*

YIELD: 4 SERVINGS

273 Cal (27% from Fat, 41% from Protein, 32% from Carb); 29 g Protein; 9 g Tot Fat; 1 g Sat Fat; 5 g Mono Fat; 22 g Carb; 6 g Fiber; 7 g Sugar; 71 mg Calcium; 2 mg Iron; 99 mg Sodium; 61 mg Cholesterol

Shrimp Scampi

FOR THE SHRIMP:

4 tablespoons olive oil

2 pounds large shrimp, shelled and deveined

2 red bell peppers, seeded, ribs removed, and sliced

4 large garlic cloves, minced

1/2 lemon with its zest set aside

2 tablespoons fresh parsley, minced

Salt and pepper to taste

FOR THE PASTA:

1/2 cup whole wheat pasta

For the pasta:

1. Cook according to package directions.

For the shrimp:

1. Heat the oil and garlic in a large pan over medium heat.
2. Add the shrimp and cook for 1 minute stirring occasionally.
3. Add the bell peppers, lemon juice, lemon peel, parsley, and season to taste. Continue to cook for two minutes or until the shrimp are cooked through, stirring occasionally.
4. Add the cooked pasta and serve immediately.

   ▶ *This dish may be refrigerated up to 2 days.*
   ▶ *I do not recommend freezing this dish.*

YIELD: 4 SERVINGS

496 Cal (32% from Fat, 41% from Protein, 26% from Carb);
52 g Protein; 18 g Tot Fat; 3 g Sat Fat; 11 g Mono Fat; 33 g Carb; 2 g Fiber; 4 g Sugar; 161 mg Calcium; 7 mg Iron; 343 mg Sodium; 345 mg Cholesterol

3 MEAT AND POULTRY

Chicken with Mushrooms

FOR THE CHICKEN:

2 teaspoons olive oil

Four 5-ounce chicken breasts (skinless)

2 shallots, minced

1 garlic clove, minced

1/4 cup Madeira

1 1/4 cup chicken stock (low-fat and low-sodium)

1 tablespoon fresh tarragon, minced

Pinch nutmeg

Cornstarch plus water

Salt and pepper

FOR THE MUSHROOMS:

2 teaspoons olive oil

1 pound wild mushrooms, cleaned and sliced

1 tablespoon fresh tarragon, minced

Salt and pepper to taste

For the chicken:

1. Heat the oil in a nonstick pan over high heat. Add the chicken and brown on both sides. Add the shallots, garlic, and Madeira, and reduce by half. Add the chicken stock, tarragon, nutmeg, and bring to a boil. Reduce heat, cover, and simmer for 10 to 15 minutes or until the chicken is cooked through.

2. Transfer the chicken breasts to a serving platter. Cover with aluminum foil to keep warm. Reduce the sauce to end up with 3/4 cup. Thicken with a little cornstarch and water. Add any rendered chicken juices and bring to a boil. Adjust seasonings and pour over the chicken.

For the vegetables:
1. Heat oil in a nonstick pan over medium heat.
2. Add the mushrooms and cook until almost cooked through.
3. Add the tarragon, season to taste, and continue to cook for a minute. Add a little sauce from the chicken and mix well.
4. Serve the chicken breasts with the mushrooms.

> ▶ *The amount of cornstarch and water mixture may vary depending on the amount of water rendered by the chicken and the reduction process. To obtain the right thickness for a sauce: Dip a spoon in the sauce, turn it over, and make a line across with your finger. Tilt the spoon. If the sauce does not run over the line, it is the perfect thickness. If it does, you need to thicken with a little cornstarch and water mixture. After adding the mixture, you will need to bring the sauce to a boil. If it gets too thick, just add a little liquid to thin out.*
> ▶ *The chicken and mushrooms may be refrigerated separately up to 5 days.*
> ▶ *Not recommended for freezing.*
> ▶ *Add a little brown sauce to emphasize the sauce flavors.*

YIELD: 4 SERVINGS

268 Cal (26% from Fat, 59% from Protein, 15% from Carb);
37 g Protein; 7 g Tot Fat; 1 g Sat Fat; 4 g Mono Fat; 10 g Carb; 2 g Fiber; 3 g Sugar; 37 mg Calcium; 2 mg Iron; 356 mg Sodium; 82 mg Cholesterol

Chicken au Citron

3 tablespoons olive oil

Four 5-ounce chicken breasts (skinless)

5 lemons

1 tablespoon fresh poultry herbs

Salt and pepper to taste

1. Juice four lemons. Mix in two tablespoons of olive oil and the herbs, and season with pepper. Place the chicken pieces in a plastic bag. Pour the lemon marinade over the chicken and refrigerate for at least one hour, rotating every 10 minutes.
2. Preheat the broiler. Remove the chicken breasts from the marinade and pat dry. Place them on a greased cookie sheet and brush a little olive oil over each breast. Broil for approximately 6 to 7 minutes on each side. Watch carefully to avoid burning. Serve immediately with lemon wedges.

   ▸ *The chicken may be refrigerated up to 5 days.*
   ▸ *The chicken may be frozen up to 1 month.*
   ▸ *This dish goes well with Zucchini and Bell Peppers with Pine Nuts.*
   ▸ *This flavored chicken can also be used for salad, sandwich, soup, or pasta dish.*

YIELD: 4 SERVINGS

245 Cal (29% from Fat, 49% from Protein, 22% from Carb);
34 g Protein; 9 g Tot Fat; 1 g Sat Fat; 5 g Mono Fat; 15 g Carb; 6 g Fiber; 0 g Sugar; 107 mg Calcium; 2 mg Iron; 97 mg Sodium; 82 mg Cholesterol

Chicken Cacciatora

2 tablespoons olive oil

One 4-pound roasting chicken, cut into serving pieces

1/4 cup chicken stock

6 ounces onions, diced (about 1 medium onion)

1 large carrot, diced

2 celery stalks, diced

1 green bell pepper, diced

2 garlic cloves, minced

1 cup diced tomatoes (can)

1 cup mushrooms, sliced

A couple of pinches dry Italian herbs

1/2 cup brown rice

Salt and pepper to taste

1. Preheat the oven to 350°F.
2. Heat a third of the oil in a large pan over high heat. Add half the chicken pieces and brown on all sides. Transfer to a large deep oven-proof pan and repeat the process with a third of the oil and remaining chicken pieces.
3. Deglaze the pan with a little chicken stock and with a whisk scrap all the particles from the bottom and side of the pan. Add liquid and particles to the chicken. Add remaining oil and slightly brown the onion.
4. Add the carrot, celery, garlic, tomatoes, mushrooms, herbs, and bring to a boil over medium heat. Season to taste and transfer to the chicken. Cover with aluminum foil and bake for 40 to 45 minutes. Serve with the rice.
5. Meanwhile, cook the brown rice according to package directions.

  ▸ *This dish may also be cooked on the stove top over very low heat.*
  ▸ *This chicken and rice may be refrigerated separately up to 5 days.*
  ▸ *This chicken and rice may be frozen separately up to 1 month.*

YIELD: 6 TO 8 SERVING S

489 Cal (56% from Fat, 29% from Protein, 15% from Carb);
35 g Protein; 30 g Tot Fat; 8 g Sat Fat; 12 g Mono Fat; 19 g Carb; 3 g Fiber; 3 g Sugar; 48 mg Calcium; 3 mg Iron; 63 mg Sodium; 170 mg Cholesterol

Stuffed Turkey Breast with Spinach and Boursin

FOR THE TURKEY:

1 tablespoon olive oil

Four 4-ounce turkey breasts

8 fresh large basil leaves

2 ounces Boursin (with garlic and herbs), divided into four portions

1 large shallot, thinly sliced

1/4 cup Chardonnay wine

1 cup chicken stock (low-fat and low-sodium)

4 pinches dry Italian herbs

2 tablespoons fresh parsley, minced

Cornstarch plus a little water

Salt and pepper to taste

FOR THE VEGETABLES:

2 pounds fresh spinach, washed and patted dry

Salt and pepper to taste

For the turkey:

1. Preheat the oven to 350 F.
2. Place the turkey breasts between two plastic wrap sheets. Flatten with a mallet until fairly thin. Sprinkle pepper and a pinch of Italian herbs on each breast. Spread one portion of Boursin, add 2 basil leaves, and roll each breast tightly. Secure with a few toothpicks so it does not unroll on its own.
3. Heat the oil in a sauté pan over high heat. Add the turkey rolls, placing the folded side down first. Brown and turn over.
4. Once browned, add the shallot, wine, and half of the chicken stock. Bring to a boil and place in the oven for 10 to 12 minutes.
5. Transfer the rolls to a serving platter and cover with aluminum foil to keep warm. Add the remaining stock to the sauce and reduce to end up with less than 1 cup. Thicken with a little cornstarch water mixture.
6. Add the parsley and any rendered turkey juices, and bring to a boil. Adjust seasonings and pour over the turkey. Serve immediately with the steamed spinach.

For the accompaniment:

1. While the sauce is reducing, preheat a steamer. Put the spinach in the steamer basket and cook until slightly wilted. Season to taste and serve

with the stuffed turkey.

▶ *The amount of cornstarch and water mixture may vary depending on the amount of water rendered by the turkey and the reduction process. To obtain the right thickness for a sauce: dip a spoon in the sauce, turn it over, and make a line across with your finger. Tilt the spoon. If the sauce does not run over the line, it is the perfect thickness. If it does, you need to thicken with a little cornstarch and water mixture. After adding the mixture, you will need to bring the sauce to a boil. If it gets too thick, just add a little liquid to thin out.*
▶ *The basil leaves may be replaced with spinach leaves.*
▶ *The turkey and spinach may be refrigerated separately up to 5 days.*
▶ *The turkey may be frozen separately up to 1 month. The spinach is best cooked just before eating.*
▶ *Add a little brown sauce to emphasize the sauce flavors.*

YIELD: 4 SERVINGS

364 Cal (41% from Fat, 46% from Protein, 13% from Carb);
42 g Protein; 16 g Tot Fat; 5 g Sat Fat; 6 g Mono Fat; 12 g Carb; 5 g Fiber; 1 g Sugar; 272 mg Calcium; 8 mg Iron; 329 mg Sodium; 95 mg Cholesterol

Turkey Breast with Sage

2 tablespoons olive oil

1 turkey breast (about 2 pounds)

1 tablespoon ground sage

3 to 4 fresh sage leaves

1/2 cup chicken stock

Cornstarch

Salt and pepper to taste

1. Preheat the oven to 350°F.
2. Mix the ground sage with a little pepper and spread all over the turkey breast under its skin. Be careful not to break the skin. Brush olive oil over the skin.
3. Place the turkey skin-side up in a roasting pan. Pour the chicken stock in the pan, add the sage leaves, and bake for an hour or until a meat thermometer registers 180°F.
4. Remove the turkey breast from the pan, cover with aluminum foil to keep warm. Remove the sage leaves from the sauce and thicken with a little cornstarch and water mixture. Adjust seasonings and serve over the turkey breast slices.

   ▸ *This dish may be refrigerated up to 5 days.*
   ▸ *This dish may be frozen up to 1 month.*
   ▸ *Use the turkey meat to make salad, sandwich, or pasta dish.*

YIELD: 4 SERVINGS

341 Cal (50% from Fat, 48% from Protein, 2% from Carb);
40 g Protein; 18 g Tot Fat; 4 g Sat Fat; 9 g Mono Fat; 1 g Carb; 0 g Fiber; 0 g Sugar; 32 mg Calcium; 2 mg Iron; 189 mg Sodium; 118 mg Cholesterol

Tuscan Beef Stew

2 tablespoons olive oil

2 pounds lean beef (stew meat)

6 ounces onions, diced (about 1 medium onion)

6 ounces celery stalks, sliced (about 3 celery stalks)

2 garlic cloves, minced

1/2 cup red Burgundy wine

2 whole cloves

2 1/2 cups diced tomatoes

3 parsley branches, minced

3 medium potatoes, quartered (about 18 ounces potatoes)

1 bouquet garni

Salt and pepper to taste

1. Heat 2 teaspoons of oil in a pan over high heat.
2. Add the onion and garlic, and sauté until translucent. Transfer to a stockpot. Using the same pan, add a little oil and brown half the meat.
3. Transfer the meat to the stockpot and repeat the process with the remaining beef. Deglaze the pan with the wine and swirl to dissolve the cooked particles on the bottom and side of the pan. Transfer the hot liquid to the stockpot.
4. Heat the stockpot over medium heat. Add the cloves, tomatoes, celery, parsley and bouquet garni, and season with pepper to taste. Cook over low heat for 1 hour.
5. Add the potatoes and continue to cook for 20 minutes. If the meat is not tender enough, remove the potatoes, and continue to cook until tender. Adjust seasonings and serve immediately.

▶ *The stew may be refrigerated up to 5 days.*
▶ *The stew may be frozen up to 1 month.*

YIELD: 8 SERVINGS

434 Cal (49% from Fat, 34% from Protein, 17% from Carb);
36 g Protein; 23 g Tot Fat; 8 g Sat Fat; 11 g Mono Fat; 18 g Carb; 3 g Fiber; 2 g Sugar; 39 mg Calcium; 5 mg Iron; 100 mg Sodium; 113 mg Cholesterol

Lamb Chops Roman Style

2 tablespoons olive oil

8 loin lamb chops (approximately 1 3/4 pounds)

2 garlic cloves, sliced

1 teaspoon freshly minced rosemary plus 2 branches

1 teaspoon dry parsley

Salt and pepper to taste

1. Slash fat around lamb chops to prevent curling during the cooking process. Brush the lamb chops with the rosemary branches. Sprinkle pepper to taste.
2. Heat the oil, garlic, and the teaspoon of minced rosemary in a large sauté pan over medium heat. As soon as it is hot, strain the oil and discard the garlic and rosemary. Sauté the lamb chops in that oil until browned on both sides (about 3 minutes on each side). Sprinkle salt to taste and parsley, and serve immediately.

▶ *This dish goes well with the Broccoli with Parmesan.*
▶ *The lamb chops may be refrigerated up to 5 days.*
▶ *The lamb chops may be frozen up to 1 month.*

YIELD: 4 SERVINGS

322 Cal (48% from Fat, 52% from Protein, 0% from Carb);
41 g Protein; 17 g Tot Fat; 5 g Sat Fat; 9 g Mono Fat; 0 g Carb; 0 g Fiber; 0 g Sugar; 20 mg Calcium; 4 mg Iron; 128 mg Sodium; 127 mg Cholesterol

VEGETABLES AND GRAINS

Baked Tomatoes Italian Style

4 large tomatoes

2 tablespoons olive oil

4 teaspoons anchovy paste

2 tablespoons garlic cloves, minced

4 large pinches freshly minced basil

1/4 cup Italian breadcrumbs

1/4 cup grated parmesan

Pepper to taste

1. Preheat the oven to 375°F.
2. Cut the tomatoes in half. On each half, spread a little anchovy paste and sprinkle 1/4 teaspoon olive oil.
3. Add garlic and pepper to taste. Sprinkle the basil, Italian breadcrumbs, and parmesan.
4. Place in a baking dish and bake for 20 to 25 minutes. Serve immediately.

▶ *Because, anchovy paste is very salty, I do not add salt in the recipe.*
▶ *The tomatoes may be refrigerated up to 2 days.*
▶ *Not recommended for freezing.*

YIELD: 4 SERVINGS

181 Cal (51% from Fat, 20% from Protein, 29% from Carb);
9 g Protein; 10 g Tot Fat; 2 g Sat Fat; 6 g Mono Fat; 14 g Carb; 2 g Fiber; 5 g Sugar; 135 mg Calcium; 2 mg Iron; 824 mg Sodium; 18 mg Cholesterol

〜∽

Broccoli with Parmesan

1 1/2 pounds broccoli florets

2 tablespoons plus 1 teaspoon olive oil

1/4 cup grated Parmesan

Salt and pepper to taste

1. Preheat the oven to 375°F.
   Bring a pan of slightly salted water to a boil. Blanch the broccoli florets for 10 seconds and immediately place them in ice cold water in order to stop the cooking process. Remove from the ice cold water and pat dry.
2. Place the broccoli florets in a greased baking dish and brush them with the 2 tablespoons of olive oil. Season to taste and sprinkle the Parmesan cheese.
3. Bake for 10 to 12 minutes or until the cheese is nicely brown. Serve immediately.

   ▸ *The blanched broccoli may be refrigerated up to 5 days.*
   ▸ *The blanched broccoli may be frozen up to 1 month.*

YIELD: 4 SERVINGS

1189 Cal (56% from Fat, 20% from Protein, 24% from Carb);
10 g Protein; 13 g Tot Fat; 4 g Sat Fat; 7 g Mono Fat; 12 g Carb; 4 g Fiber; 3 g Sugar; 237 mg Calcium; 1 mg Iron; 273 mg Sodium; 12 mg Cholesterol

$\sim$

Zucchini and Bell Peppers
with Pine Nuts

1 tablespoon olive oil

4 ounces onions, sliced (about 1 small onion)

12 ounces zucchini, sliced (about 2 zucchini)

12 ounces red bell peppers, sliced (about 2 bell peppers)

1/4 cup pine nuts

2 pinches dry Italian herbs

Salt and pepper to taste

1. Heat the oil in a large pan over high heat.
2. Add the onion and sauté until translucent.
3. Add the zucchini, bell peppers, and herbs, and sauté until slightly browned and cooked through over medium heat. Mix occasionally to avoid burning.
4. Add the pine nuts and season to taste.

   ▸ *The vegetables may be refrigerated up to 5 days.*
   ▸ *The vegetables may be frozen up to 1 month.*

YIELD: 4 SERVINGS

117 Cal (66% from Fat, 9% from Protein, 25% from Carb);
3 g Protein; 9 g Tot Fat; 1 g Sat Fat; 4 g Mono Fat; 8 g Carb; 3 g Fiber; 4 g Sugar; 23 mg Calcium; 1 mg Iron; 11 mg Sodium; 0 mg Cholesterol

~~

Eggplant Provençal
with Pecorino Shavings

1 tablespoon olive oil

1 small onion, sliced (about 4 ounces onion)

1 eggplant, skin removed and diced (about 10 ounces eggplant)

2 garlic cloves, minced

1 tomato (about 6 ounces tomato)

2 pinches herbs de Provence

1/4 cup pecorino shavings

Salt and pepper to taste

1. Make a small X incision on the top and bottom of the tomato. Blanch the tomato for 20 seconds. Place immediately in ice-cold water to stop the cooking process. Peel, seed, and dice the tomato.
2. Heat the oil in a large pan over high heat.
3. Add the onion and sauté until translucent.
4. Add the eggplant and herbs, and continue to cook over low heat until slightly tender, mixing occasionally.
5. Mix in the garlic and tomato, and continue to cook until the eggplant is very tender. Season to taste and transfer to a serving platter. Sprinkle with the Pecorino shavings and serve immediately.

> ▸ *The vegetables may be refrigerated without the cheese up to 5 days.*
> ▸ *The vegetables may be frozen without the cheese up to 1 month.*

YIELD: 4 SERVINGS

97 Cal (47% from Fat, 15% from Protein, 37% from Carb);
4 g Protein; 5 g Tot Fat; 2 g Sat Fat; 3 g Mono Fat; 10 g Carb; 4 g Fiber; 4 g Sugar; 87 mg
Calcium; 0 mg Iron; 100 mg Sodium; 6 mg Cholesterol

Spinach with Walnuts and Balsamic Vinegar

6 cups fresh spinach

4 tablespoons olive oil

2 tablespoons balsamic vinegar

Pinch of nutmeg

1/4 cup walnuts, chopped

Salt and pepper to taste

1. Mix the 3 tablespoons of olive oil, balsamic vinegar, and nutmeg in a large bowl. Season to taste and set aside.
2. Heat 1 1/2 teaspoon of olive oil in a large skillet over medium heat.
3. Add half of the spinach and quickly sauté until barely wilted. Transfer the spinach to a platter.
4. Heat the remaining oil and spinach and sauté until barely wilted. Add the first batch to the pan and blend in the vinaigrette. Transfer to a serving platter, sprinkle with the walnuts, and serve immediately.

YIELD: 4 SERVINGS

178 Cal (88% from Fat, 5% from Protein, 6% from Carb);
2 g Protein; 18 g Tot Fat; 2 g Sat Fat; 11 g Mono Fat; 3 g Carb; 1 g Fiber; 1 g Sugar; 52 mg Calcium; 2 mg Iron; 36 mg Sodium; 0 mg Cholesterol

~~

Green Beans with Mushrooms

1 1/2 tablespoon olive oil

4 ounces onions, sliced (about 1 small onion)

1 pound green beans, ends trimmed

1/2 cup mushrooms, sliced

2 garlic cloves, minced

2 pinches fresh thyme, minced

2 tablespoons fresh basil, minced

1 tablespoon fresh parsley, minced

Salt and pepper to taste

1. Place the green beans in a large pan and fill with enough water to cover them. Add 1 teaspoon of salt and bring to boil over high heat. Reduce heat and simmer until tender. Drain and set aside.
2. Heat 1 tablespoon of oil in a nonstick pan over medium heat.
3. Add the onion and sauté until translucent.
4. Add the garlic, mushrooms, and herbs, and sauté for 2 minutes. Blend in the green beans and remaining oil. Season to taste and serve immediately.

   ▶ This dish may be refrigerated up to 2 days.
   ▶ This dish may be frozen up to 1 month.

YIELD: 4 SERVINGS

94 Cal (46% from Fat, 10% from Protein, 44% from Carb);
3 g Protein; 5 g Tot Fat; 1 g Sat Fat; 4 g Mono Fat; 11 g Carb; 4 g Fiber; 3 g Sugar; 52 mg
Calcium; 1 mg Iron; 9 mg Sodium; 0 mg Cholesterol

Brown Rice Pilaf

1 cup brown rice

2 teaspoons olive oil

12 ounces onions, diced small (about 2 medium onions)

6 ounces carrots, diced small (about 2 medium carrots)

6 ounces yellow bell peppers, diced small (about 1 medium bell pepper)

1 garlic clove, minced

2 1/4 cups vegetable stock

2 tablespoons fresh parsley, minced

Salt and pepper to taste

1. Rinse the rice twice and drain.
2. Heat the oil in a deep pan over high heat.
3. Add the vegetables and sauté for 2 minutes.
4. Add the rice and sauté for a minute.
5. Add the stock and parsley, and bring to a boil. Cover, reduce heat, and cook until tender (approximately 40 minutes but it may depend of the type of rice you use; for best result, see package instructions). Adjust seasonings and remove from heat. Strain if necessary, and serve immediately.

   ▶ *You may add fresh herbs based on the accompaniment flavor.*
   ▶ *This rice may be refrigerated for 5 days.*
   ▶ *This rice may be frozen for 1 month.*

YIELD: 8 SERVINGS

134 Cal (6% from Fat, 9% from Protein, 84% from Carb);
3 g Protein; 1 g Tot Fat; 0 g Sat Fat; 0 g Mono Fat; 29 g Carb; 2 g Fiber; 4 g Sugar; 43 mg Calcium; 1 mg Iron; 55 mg Sodium; 0 mg Cholesterol

~

Pasta with Vegetables
and Sundried Tomatoes

8 ounces wheat penne

4 teaspoons olive oil

2 ounces onions, diced (about 1/2 small onion)

6 ounces yellow bell peppers, diced (about 1 medium bell pepper)

8 ounces broccoli florets

2 garlic cloves, minced

10 sundried tomatoes packed in oil, julienned

1/4 teaspoon red pepper flakes

2 tablespoons pine nuts

A bunch of fresh basil leaves, julienned

1/4 cup grated parmesan

Salt and pepper to taste

1. Bring a pan of slightly salted water plus 1 teaspoon of olive oil to a boil. Add the penne and cook until al dente, about 10 to 12 minutes. Drain and return to the pan. Mix in 1 teaspoon of olive oil.
2. Heat 2 teaspoons of olive oil in a pan over high heat.
3. Add the onions and sauté until translucent.
4. Add the bell peppers and garlic, and cook for 2 minutes, mixing occasionally.
5. Add the broccoli and sundried tomatoes, and continue to cook until the vegetables are tender. Add a little bit of the oil from the sundried tomatoes, the pine nuts, and basil, and season to taste. Blend in the cooked pasta and serve immediately.

▸ *This dish may be refrigerated up to 5 days.*
▸ *This dish may be frozen up to 1 month.*

YIELD: 4 SERVINGS

347 Cal (29% from Fat, 11% from Protein, 60% from Carb);
10 g Protein; 12 g Tot Fat; 2 g Sat Fat; 6 g Mono Fat; 55 g Carb; 7 g Fiber; 1 g Sugar; 111 mg Calcium; 2 mg Iron; 134 mg Sodium; 6 mg Cholesterol

Macaroni and Cheese à la Française

8 ounces whole wheat macaroni

2 tablespoons butter

4 ounces Gruyère cheese, finely shredded

1/4 cup low-fat milk, hot (2% milk)

Pinch of nutmeg

Salt and pepper to taste

1. Bring a pan of slightly salted water plus 1 teaspoon of canola oil to a boil.
2. Add the macaroni and cook until al dente. Please refer to package instructions for more information on cooking time. Drain and return to the hot pan.
3. Over very low heat, mix in the butter, Gruyère, and milk. Continue to mix until the cheese is melted.
4. Remove from heat, add a pinch of nutmeg, and season to taste. Serve immediately.

> ▶ *The dish may be refrigerated up to 3 days.*
> ▶ *This dish is not recommended for freezing.*
> ▶ *You may replace the butter with vegetable oil for a healthier choice.*
> ▶ *Gruyère cheese is what makes this dish unique. However, if not available, you may substitute Swiss cheese.*
> ▶ *Serve with vegetables on the side or a small vegetables salad.*
> ▶ *You can also mix with the pasta a small amount of diced vegetables, ground cooked turkey, diced pieces of cooked white meat, salmon, or tuna.*
> ▶ *You may remove or add more cheese. Just keep in mind that Gruyère cheese has the calories shown below.*

YIELD: 4 SERVINGS

1 ounce Gruyère: 117 Cal (71% from Fat, 29% from Protein, 0% from Carb); 8 g Protein; 9 g Tot Fat; 5 g Sat Fat; 3 g Mono Fat; 0 g Carb; 0 g Fiber; 0 g Sugar; 287 mg Calcium; 0 mg Iron; 95 mg Sodium; 31 mg Cholesterol

---

YIELD: 6 SERVINGS

For the above recipe and per serving: 170 Cal (55% from Fat, 18% from Protein, 27% from Carb); 8 g Protein; 10 g Tot Fat; 6 g Sat Fat; 3 g Mono Fat; 11 g Carb; 0 g Fiber; 1 g Sugar; 207 mg Calcium; 0 mg Iron; 69 mg Sodium; 32 mg Cholesterol
Serving size: 4 ounces cooked pasta

5
SOUPS AND SALADS

Carrot and Thyme Soup

1 teaspoon canola oil

4 ounces onions, minced

1 pound carrots, shredded

1 garlic clove, minced

1/2 cup vegetable stock (low-fat and low-sodium)

3 ounces potatoes, skin removed and shredded (about 1 small potato)

1/2 tablespoon honey

1 teaspoon fresh minced thyme

1 bay leaf

1 teaspoon vanilla extract

1/4 cup low-fat milk, hot

Salt and pepper to taste

1. Heat the oil in a large pan over high heat.
2. Add the onions and sauté until translucent.
3. Add the carrots and garlic, and cook for 1 minute.
4. Add the stock, potatoes, honey, thyme, and bay leaf, and bring to a boil.
5. Reduce heat, cover, and simmer for 15 minutes. Remove the bay leaf.
6. Purée the soup in a blender and return to pan.
7. Add the vanilla and hot milk, and bring to a boil over medium heat. Swirl with a spoon to prevent burning. Season to taste and serve immediately.

   ▶ *The soup may be refrigerated up to 3 days.*
   ▶ *The soup may be frozen up to 1 month.*
   ▶ *Vegetable stock may be replaced with chicken stock.*

YIELD: 4 SERVINGS

112 Cal (16% from Fat, 9% from Protein, 76% from Carb);
2 g Protein; 2 g Tot Fat; 0 g Sat Fat; 1 g Mono Fat; 22 g Carb; 4 g Fiber; 10 g Sugar; 70 mg
Calcium; 1 mg Iron; 103 mg Sodium; 2 mg Cholesterol

Mushroom and Barley Soup

2 teaspoons canola oil

2 ounces barley (uncooked)

6 ounces onions, diced small (about 1 medium onion)

4 ounces carrots, diced small (about 1 large carrot)

6 ounces turnips, diced (about 1 medium turnip)

5 cups chicken stock (low-fat and low-sodium)

1 bouquet garni

8 ounces mushrooms, diced (about 8 white mushrooms)

2 tablespoons fresh parsley, minced

Salt and pepper to taste

1. Cook the barley according to package directions. Drain and set aside.
2. Heat the oil in a pan over high heat.
3. Add the onion, carrot, and turnip, and sauté for 2 minutes.
4. Add the stock and bouquet garni, and bring to a boil. Reduce heat and simmer until the vegetables are barely tender (about 10 minutes).
5. Add the mushrooms and cooked barley, and bring to a simmer. Continue to cook for another 5 minutes. Add parsley and season to taste.

   ▸ *The soup may be refrigerated up to 5 days.*
   ▸ *The soup may be frozen up to 1 month.*
   ▸ *Chicken stock can be replaced with vegetable stock.*

YIELD: 4 TO 6 SERVINGS

257 Cal (33% from Fat, 10% from Protein, 56% from Carb);
7 g Protein; 10 g Tot Fat; 1 g Sat Fat; 5 g Mono Fat; 38 g Carb; 7 g Fiber; 9 g Sugar; 61 mg Calcium; 3 mg Iron; 1056 mg Sodium; 0 mg Cholesterol

⟡

Spinach and Onion Soup

2 tablespoons olive oil

6 ounces onions, thinly sliced (about 1 medium onion)

12 ounces fresh baby spinach leaves, washed and patted dry

12 ounces potatoes, thinly sliced

1 bunch fresh tarragon, chopped

1 bunch fresh chervil, chopped

5 to 6 cups beef stock (low-fat and low-sodium)

4 tablespoon cream, hot (option)

Salt and pepper

1. Heat the oil in a large pan over medium heat.
2. Add the onions and cook until translucent.
3. Add the spinach, potatoes, and stock, and bring to a boil. Reduce heat and cook for 20 minutes uncovered.
4. Add the herbs, adjust seasonings, and continue to cook for another 5 minutes.
5. Add the hot cream, bring to a boil, and serve immediately.

▶ *The soup may be refrigerated up to 2 days.*
▶ *The soup may be frozen up to 1 month.*
▶ *Beef stock can be replaced with vegetable stock.*

YIELD: 4 SERVINGS

197 Cal (43% from Fat, 9% from Protein, 48% from Carb);
5 g Protein; 10 g Tot Fat; 3 g Sat Fat; 6 g Mono Fat; 25 g Carb; 4 g Fiber; 3 g Sugar; 103 mg Calcium; 3 mg Iron; 75 mg Sodium; 10 mg Cholesterol

Pumpkin Soup and Pepitas

1 teaspoon olive oil

6 ounces onions, minced (about 1 medium onion)

2 garlic cloves, minced

3 cups chicken stock (low-fat and low-sodium)

One 15-ounce can unflavored pumpkin purée

1 1/2 cup low-fat evaporated milk

1 teaspoon vanilla

2 fresh sage leaves

2 tablespoons pepitas

Salt and pepper to taste

1. Heat the oil in a large pan over medium heat.
2. Add the onions and sauté until translucent.
3. Stir in the garlic and continue to cook for another minute.
4. Add the pumpkin puree, stock, and sage. Mix occasionally while bringing to a boil.
5. Add the evaporated milk and vanilla, and bring to a boil, still stirring occasionally. Season to taste and garnish with the pepitas before serving.

   ▸ *The soup may be refrigerated up to 2 days.*
   ▸ *The soup may be frozen up to 1 month.*

YIELD: 4 TO 6 SERVINGS

178 Cal (22% from Fat, 19% from Protein, 59% from Carb);
9 g Protein; 4 g Tot Fat; 1 g Sat Fat; 2 g Mono Fat; 27 g Carb; 4 g Fiber; 15 g Sugar; 267 mg Calcium; 2 mg Iron; 587 mg Sodium; 3 mg Cholesterol

Bean Soup

2 teaspoons canola oil

8 ounces onions, diced small (about 1 large onion)

4 ounces carrots, diced small (about 1 large carrot)

4 ounces celery stalks, diced small (about 2 large celery stalks)

2 garlic cloves, minced

6 cups chicken stock (low-fat and low-sodium)

12 ounces dried black beans, rinsed

1 bouquet garni

Salt and pepper to taste

1. Place the beans in a large pot and cover (way over) with water. Bring to a boil over high heat. Remove from heat and let soak for an hour. Or you may soak the beans overnight in cold water. Strain and set aside.
2. Heat the oil in a large pan over high heat.
3. Add the onions and sauté until translucent.
4. Add the carrot, celery, stock, and garlic, and cook for 2 minutes.
5. Add the beans, bouquet garni, and bring to a boil.
6. Reduce heat, cover, and simmer for 45 minutes or until tender. Skim the surface as needed.
7. Remove 1/3 cup of the bean and purée with a fork. Mix the puree with the remaining soup. Remove the bouquet garni, adjust seasonings and serve immediately. If the soup is too thick, adjust with stock. If the soup is too thin, reduce the liquid more.

   ▸ *The soup may be refrigerated up to 5 days.*
   ▸ *The soup may be frozen up to 1 month.*
   ▸ *Chicken stock may be replaced with vegetable stock.*

YIELD: 4 TO 6 SERVINGS

198 Cal (13% from Fat, 26% from Protein, 61% from Carb);
13 g Protein; 3 g Tot Fat; 0 g Sat Fat; 1 g Mono Fat; 31 g Carb; 10 g Fiber; 4 g Sugar; 86 mg Calcium; 3 mg Iron; 877 mg Sodium; 0 mg Cholesterol

Tom Soup

4 teaspoons olive oil

Four 4-ounce white fish fillets

2 leeks, cleaned and diced medium

6 garlic cloves, minced

One 15-ounce can diced tomato (no salt added)

1 1/2 cups diced potato (uncooked)

5 cups vegetable stock

A few saffron threads

1 bouquet garni

Salt and pepper to taste

1. Preheat the broiler. Heat 2 teaspoons of oil in a large pan over high heat.
2. Add the leeks and garlic, and sauté for 2 minutes.
3. Add the tomatoes, potatoes, saffron, stock, and bouquet garni, and simmer until the vegetables are very tender.
4. Remove bouquet garni and puree with a food mill or hand mixer. If needed, continue to reduce over low-medium heat to reach a creamy consistency. Taste and adjust seasonings. Remove from heat and cover to keep warm.
5. Place the fish fillets on a parchment paper on a cookie sheet and rub 2 teaspoons olive oil all over the fillets. Sprinkle with salt and pepper to taste. Place under the broiler and cook until the fillets become flaky (about 5 to 6 minutes or so based on thickness).
6. If necessary, reheat the soup base a bit. Serve the soup in individual bowl. Crumble one fish fillet over each bowl and serve immediately.

▶ *This dish may be refrigerated up to 2 days, keeping the fish separated.*
▶ *This dish may be frozen up to 1 month, keeping the fish separated.*

YIELD: 4 SERVINGS

343 Cal (20% from Fat, 37% from Protein, 44% from Carb);
33 g Protein; 8 g Tot Fat; 2 g Sat Fat; 4 g Mono Fat; 38 g Carb; 4 g Fiber; 8 g Sugar; 127 mg Calcium; 3 mg Iron; 304 mg Sodium; 77 mg Cholesterol

Lentil Soup with Ground Turkey

3 teaspoons canola oil

8 ounces onions, diced small (about 1 large onion)

4 ounces carrots, diced small (about 1 large carrot)

4 ounces celery stalks, diced small (about 2 large celery stalks)

2 garlic cloves, minced

6 cups chicken stock (low-fat and low-sodium)

12 ounces dried lentils (about 3 cups)

8 ounces ground turkey

1 bouquet garni

Salt and pepper

1. Heat 2 teaspoons of oil in a large pan over high heat.
2. Add the onions and sauté until translucent.
3. Add the carrot, celery, and garlic, and cook for 2 minutes.
4. Add the stock, lentils, bouquet garni, and bring to a boil.
5. Reduce heat, cover, and simmer for 35 minutes. Skim the surface as needed. Continue to simmer uncovered for 10 minutes in order to thicken the soup. Remove the bouquet garni.
6. Heat 1 teaspoon of oil in a medium pan over high heat. Add the ground turkey and sauté until cooked through (about 3 to 4 minutes). Strain and discard any fat. Add the meat to the prepared lentils and bring to a boil. Adjust seasonings and serve immediately.
7. If the soup is too thick, dilute with stock. If the soup is too thin, reduce the liquid more or mash a little bit of the lentils and return mixture to the pan.

▶ *The soup may be refrigerated up to 5 days.*
▶ *The soup may be frozen up to 1 month.*
▶ *Chicken stock may be replaced with vegetable stock.*

YIELD: 4 TO 6 SERVINGS

262 Cal (19% from Fat, 39% from Protein, 42% from Carb);
26 g Protein; 6 g Tot Fat; 1 g Sat Fat; 2 g Mono Fat; 28 g Carb; 9 g Fiber; 6 g Sugar; 87 mg Calcium; 5 mg Iron; 917 mg Sodium; 37 mg Cholesterol

Beet Salad

FOR THE SALAD:

3 medium red beets (about 2 pounds)

6 ounces golden delicious apples (about 1 medium apple)

1/4 cup walnuts, chopped

1 tablespoon raisins

FOR THE DRESSING:

2 ounces sweet onions, minced

1 garlic clove, crushed and pureed

3 tablespoons walnut oil

2 tablespoons cider vinegar

1 tablespoon fresh parsley, minced

Salt and pepper to taste

For the dressing:
1. In a bowl mix the onion, garlic, oil, vinegar, and parsley.

For the salad:
1. Wash the beets and pat dry. Remove skin and shred the beets over a bowl. Be careful because beet juice stains clothing. Peel and core the apple. Shred and add to the shredded beets.
2. Mix the beet mixture with the dressing, season to taste, and refrigerate for an hour. Sprinkle with the walnut, add the raisins, and serve immediately.

> ▶ *Try thinly slicing the beets and apple for a different look and texture.*

YIELD: 4 SERVINGS

278 Cal (47% from Fat, 7% from Protein, 46% from Carb); 5 g Protein; 15 g Tot Fat; 1 g Sat Fat; 3 g Mono Fat; 34 g Carb; 8 g Fiber; 23 g Sugar; 55 mg Calcium; 2 mg Iron; 179 mg Sodium; 0 mg Cholesterol

Belgian Endive
with Gorgonzola and Walnut

FOR THE SALAD:

1 pound Belgian endives (about 6 Belgium endives)

1/4 cup walnuts, chopped

2 ounces Gorgonzola

FOR THE DRESSING:

2 tablespoons walnut oil

1 tablespoon red wine vinegar

1 tablespoon milk mixed with a dash of mashed Gorgonzola

1 tablespoon fresh salad herbs, chopped

Salt and pepper to taste

For the dressing:
1. Mix the oil, vinegar, and milk mixture. Add herbs and season to taste.

For the salad:
1. Slice the endives. Discard the trunk of each endive.
2. Wash and dry the endives with a salad spinner. Transfer to a bowl and mix with the dressing.
3. Add the walnuts and the crumbled remaining Gorgonzola. Toss lightly and serve immediately.

YIELD: 4 SERVINGS

198 Cal (72% from Fat, 15% from Protein, 14% from Carb);
8 g Protein; 17 g Tot Fat; 4 g Sat Fat; 4 g Mono Fat; 7 g Carb; 6 g Fiber; 1 g Sugar; 244 mg Calcium; 2 mg Iron; 87 mg Sodium; 16 mg Cholesterol

Artichoke and Tomato Salad

FOR THE SALAD:

1 cup cooked artichoke hearts

12 ounces tomatoes, quartered (about 2 large tomatoes)

4 ounces Boston lettuce

FOR THE VINAIGRETTE:

1 shallot, minced

1 large garlic clove, minced

1 teaspoon Dijon mustard

2 tablespoons balsamic vinegar

4 tablespoons olive oil

1 tablespoon fresh salad herbs, minced

1 tablespoon fresh basil, minced

Salt and pepper to taste

For the vinaigrette:
1. In a bowl mix the shallot, garlic, mustard, and vinegar. Slowly whisk in the oil.
2. Add the herbs and season to taste.

For the salad:
1. Place the artichoke hearts and tomatoes in a bowl. Add half of the dressing and toss carefully.
2. In a bowl mix the lettuce with the remaining dressing and equally divide among four plates.
3. Top with the artichoke hearts and tomatoes.

YIELD: 4 SERVINGS

163 Cal (73% from Fat, 6% from Protein, 21% from Carb);
3 g Protein; 14 g Tot Fat; 2 g Sat Fat; 10 g Mono Fat; 9 g Carb; 3 g Fiber; 1 g Sugar; 27 mg Calcium; 1 mg Iron; 53 mg Sodium; 0 mg Cholesterol

Four Bean Salad

FOR THE SALAD:

8 ounces dried garbanzo beans

8 ounces dried black beans

8 ounces dried red beans

8 ounces green beans

2 ounces red onions, diced (about 1/2 small red onion)

FOR THE DRESSING:

1 large garlic clove, minced

4 tablespoons olive oil

9 tablespoons white balsamic vinegar

3 to 4 tablespoon fresh salad herbs, minced

Salt and pepper to taste

For the dressing:
1. In a bowl mix the garlic, oil, vinegar, and herbs.

For the salad:
1. Cook the beans separately following the packages instructions. Generally, it takes about 30 to 45 minutes to cook these types of beans.
2. Place the green beans with a little salt in a pan and bring to boil over high heat. Cook to desired tenderness. Strain and place immediately in ice-cold water to stop the cooking process. Strain and pat dry.
3. Place all the beans and red onion in a large bowl. Add the dressing, season to taste, and refrigerate for an hour before serving.

   ▶ *Option: This salad may be served over lettuce, rice, and/or tomatoes.*
   ▶ *You may substitute one 15-ounce can cooked beans for each type of dried bean. Rinse before use.*

YIELD: 12 SERVINGS

245 Cal (22% from Fat, 20% from Protein, 58% from Carb); 13 g Protein; 6 g Tot Fat; 1 g Sat Fat; 4 g Mono Fat; 37 g Carb; 12 g Fiber; 4 g Sugar; 79 mg Calcium; 4 mg Iron; 12 mg Sodium; 0 mg Cholesterol

Chicken Salad with Fruit

FOR THE SALAD:

5 ounces fresh spinach

8 ounces cooked chicken breasts (without skin), diced

2 avocados, diced

6 ounces red grapes

1 orange, cut into wedges

1 mango, diced

4 teaspoons sliced almonds

FOR THE DRESSING:

2 tablespoons olive oil

2 tablespoons lemon juice

1 tablespoon fresh salad herbs

Pinch of each curry and ginger

Salt and pepper to taste

For the dressing:
1. In a bowl mix the oil, lemon, and herbs.
2. Blend in the curry and ginger, and season to taste.

For the salad:
1. In a bowl mix the spinach, chicken, and dressing.
2. Add the fruit, avocados, and almonds.

YIELD: 4 SERVINGS

376 Cal (51% from Fat, 17% from Protein, 32% from Carb); 17 g Protein; 22 g Tot Fat; 3 g Sat Fat; 15 g Mono Fat; 32 g Carb; 9 g Fiber; 19 g Sugar; 89 mg Calcium; 2 mg Iron; 75 mg Sodium; 33 mg Cholesterol

Salade Niçoise au Citron

FOR THE SALAD:

5 ounces mesclun

6 ounces canned tuna in water, strained

2 large tomatoes, seeded and diced

1 yellow bell pepper, seeded, ribs removed, and julienned

1 small cucumber, peeled and sliced

4 ounces cooked green beans, cut in half

2 ounces small niçoise black olives

4 anchovies

4 eggs

FOR THE DRESSING:

1 shallot, minced

1 garlic clove, minced

3 tablespoons lemon juice

3 tablespoons olive oil

2 tablespoons salad herbs

Salt and pepper to taste

For the dressing:
1. In a bowl mix the shallot, garlic, lemon juice, oil, 1 tablespoon of herbs, and season to taste.

For the salad:
1. Place the eggs in a pan, cover with water, add 2 teaspoons salt, and bring to a boil over medium heat. Reduce heat and simmer for 10 minutes. Remove the eggs and place them in cold water. Peel, quarter, and set aside.
2. In a large bowl, mix the mesclun with half of the dressing. Add the tomatoes, bell peppers, cucumber, and green beans.
3. Top with the tuna, eggs and anchovies, and sprinkle with the remaining herbs. Drizzle with the remaining dressing and serve immediately.

YIELD: 4 SERVINGS

489 Cal (52% from Fat, 23% from Protein, 25% from Carb);
28 g Protein; 29 g Tot Fat; 6 g Sat Fat; 16 g Mono Fat; 32 g Carb; 5 g Fiber; 2 g Sugar;
116 mg Calcium; 5 mg Iron; 622 mg Sodium; 274 mg Cholesterol

Salmon and Asparagus Salad

FOR THE SALAD:

1 1/2 pound asparagus

8 ounces smoked salmon slices

1 lemon, cut into 4 wedges

FOR THE DRESSING:

1 teaspoon Dijon mustard

1 teaspoon honey

2 tablespoons wine vinegar

6 tablespoons olive oil

1 teaspoon fresh dill, minced

Salt and pepper

For the dressing:
1. In a bowl mix the mustard, honey, vinegar, oil, and dill, and season to taste.

For the salad:
1. Preheat a steamer. Trim the asparagus and place them in the steamer basket. Cook until barely tender. Transfer the asparagus to a bowl and mix in half of the dressing. Let cool and refrigerate until completely cold.
2. Equally divide the asparagus among four plates.
3. Top with the salmon slices and drizzle with the remaining dressing. Serve immediately with the lemon wedges.

YIELD: 4 SERVINGS

293 Cal (67% from Fat, 19% from Protein, 15% from Carb);
15 g Protein; 23 g Tot Fat; 3 g Sat Fat; 16 g Mono Fat; 12 g Carb; 5 g Fiber; 5 g Sugar; 69 mg Calcium; 5 mg Iron; 465 mg Sodium; 13 mg Cholesterol

SNACKS AND DESSERTS

6

Olive Paste and Tomato Bruschetta

FOR THE BREAD:

1 French baguette

FOR THE BRUSCHETTA

1 1/2 cups pitted black olives

2 ounces capers, rinsed
   and patted dry

4 large garlic cloves, minced

1/2 lemon, juiced

1/2 cup olive oil

2 ounces anchovy fillets, rinsed
   and patted dry

24 tomato slices (approximately 6
   large tomatoes)

24 basil leaves

Salt and pepper to taste

1. In a food processor puree the olives, capers, garlic, lemon juice, oil, and anchovy fillets. The paste should be smooth and spreadable. If it is too thick, add a little olive oil. Season to taste and refrigerate for 30 minutes.
2. Cut the baguette with a serrated knife into 3/4-inch thick slices. Place the slices on a baking sheet. Broil until golden brown. Cool before use.
3. Spread some olive paste on each bread slice and top with 1 basil leaf and 1 tomato slice. Drizzle a little olive oil over the tomato and serve immediately.

   ▶ *The paste may be refrigerated up to 5 days. Cover the paste with a thin layer of olive oil to avoid dryness.*

YIELD: 24 BRUSCHETTA

68 Cal (74% from Fat, 7% from Protein, 19% from Carb);
1 g Protein; 6 g Tot Fat; 1 g Sat Fat; 4 g Mono Fat; 3 g Carb; 1 g Fiber; 0 g Sugar; 17 mg
Calcium; 1 mg Iron; 242 mg Sodium; 2 mg Cholesterol

Spinach and Mozzarella Bruschetta

FOR THE BRUSCHETTA

2 pounds baby spinach

6 garlic cloves, cut in half lengthwise

8 ounces fresh mozzarella, diced small

12 sun-dried tomatoes packed in olive oil, diced small

2 tablespoons olive oil

1 tablespoon balsamic vinegar

Salt and pepper to taste

FOR THE BREAD

1 French baguette

1. Wash the spinach leaves and remove excess water with a salad spinner.
2. Chop coarsely and preheat a large skillet with a little olive oil.
3. Add half the spinach and sauté until slightly wilted (approximately 1 to 2 minutes), stirring constantly. Transfer the spinach to a bowl and repeat the process with the remaining spinach. Cool and discard any rendered liquid.
4. Mix in the mozzarella and the diced sun-dried tomatoes.
5. Add 1 tablespoon of the oil from the sundried tomatoes jar, 2 tablespoons of olive oil, and the balsamic vinegar. Season to taste and refrigerate for 15 minutes.
6. Preheat the broiler. With a serrated knife, cut the baguette into 1/2 inch thick slices. Place the slices on a baking sheet. Broil until golden brown. Rub each warm slice with garlic clove half. Spoon some bruschetta mixture over each slice (on garlic side) and serve immediately.

YIELD: 24 BRUSCHETTA

55 Cal (56% from Fat, 25% from Protein, 19% from Carb);
4 g Protein; 4 g Tot Fat; 1 g Sat Fat; 2 g Mono Fat; 3 g Carb; 1 g Fiber; 0 g Sugar; 113 mg Calcium; 1 mg Iron; 101 mg Sodium; 6 mg Cholesterol

Pear and Almond Bruschetta

FOR THE BRUSCHETTA

6 large pears, washed and patted dried

1/2 cup almond butter

1/4 cup sliced almonds

8 tablespoons apricot preserves

1 lemon, juiced

FOR THE BREAD:

1 country bread loaf or multi-grain bread loaf

1. Peel, core, and quarter the pears. Slice each quarter into 3 slices. Place the pears in a bowl and mix in the lemon juice to prevent browning.
2. Preheat the broiler. Cut the bread with a serrated knife into 3/4-inch thick slices. Cut each slice in half again. Place the slices on a baking sheet. Broil until golden brown. Cool before use.
3. Spread 1 teaspoon almond butter over each bread slice and top with 3 pears slices. Spread a little warmed preserves with a knife over the pear slices and sprinkle with 1/2 teaspoon sliced almonds. Serve immediately.

YIELD: 24 BRUSCHETTA

94 Cal (34% from Fat, 5% from Protein, 61% from Carb); 1 g Protein; 4 g Tot Fat; 0 g Sat Fat; 2 g Mono Fat; 15 g Carb; 2 g Fiber; 9 g Sugar; 27 mg Calcium; 0 mg Iron; 4 mg Sodium; 0 mg Cholesterol

Zucchini Stuffed with Tuna

4 green zucchinis, approximately seven inches long

18 ounces canned tuna in water

3 tablespoons fresh parsley, minced

3 tablespoons fresh chives, minced

1/3 cup scallions, chopped small

1 lemon

8 tablespoons low-fat canola mayonnaise

Fresh minced parsley

Salt and pepper to taste

1. In a bowl mix the tuna, parsley, chives, and scallions. Sprinkle a little bit of lemon juice. Mix in the mayonnaise and season to taste. Refrigerate until needed.
2. Cut off both ends of the zucchinis. Divide each zucchini into three sections. Cut each section in half lengthwise. Remove a little bit of the flesh from each zucchini center with a melon baller. You should end up with 24 pieces.
3. Parboil them for one minute in boiling salted water. Immediately place the zucchinis in ice-cold water, strain, and pat dry.
4. Top each piece with the tuna mixture, sprinkle with parsley, and serve immediately.

▶ *The tuna mixture may be refrigerated up to 2 days.*

YIELD: 24 ZUCCHINI SECTIONS

44 Cal (32% from Fat, 48% from Protein, 20% from Carb);
5 g Protein; 2 g Tot Fat; 0 g Sat Fat; 0 g Mono Fat; 2 g Carb; 1 g Fiber; 1 g Sugar; 12 mg Calcium; 0 mg Iron; 89 mg Sodium; 10 mg Cholesterol

Winter Fruit Salad

1 small banana, sliced

1 pear, diced

1 apple, diced

6 ounces grapes

1 orange, peeled and segmented

1/4 cup pomegranate seeds

2 tablespoons lemon juice

1 teaspoon vanilla extract

1. Blend all the fruits in a large bowl. Mix in the lemon juice, vanilla extract, and pomegranate seeds and refrigerate until use.

   ▸ *The salad may be refrigerated up to 2 days.*

YIELD: 4 SERVINGS

135 Cal (2% from Fat, 4% from Protein, 94% from Carb);
1 g Protein; 0 g Tot Fat; 0 g Sat Fat; 0 g Mono Fat; 35 g Carb; 4 g Fiber; 25 g Sugar; 31 mg Calcium; 0 mg Iron; 3 mg Sodium; 0 mg Cholesterol

Acai and Berries Popsicles

4 ounces pure Acai, no sugar added

4 ounces berries

4 ounces banana (about 1 small banana, skin removed)

4 ounces apple juice

1. Place all the fruits in a blender and puree on high speed. Divide
    equally among 4 popsicles maker and freeze.

    ▸ *Acai is a fruit grown in the Amazon rain forest. It has a chocolaty flavor and is
    considered to be one of nature's healthiest foods. Due to its high concentration
    of antioxidants, anthocyanins (approximately 20 times the amount in red
    wine), amino acids, essential omegas, fibers and protein, it is a great addition
    to a healthy diet.*

    ▸ *If not available in your local stores, check the Internet for this product. You
    may replace acai with Noni or Gac juice.*

    ▸ *You may keep the popsicles frozen up to a month.*

YIELD: 4 POPSICLES

76 Cal (22% from Fat, 6% from Protein, 72% from Carb);
1 g Protein; 2 g Tot Fat; 0 g Sat Fat; 0 g Mono Fat; 15 g Carb; 3 g Fiber; 8 g Sugar; 10 mg
Calcium; 0 mg Iron; 5 mg Sodium; 0 mg Cholesterol

Chocolate Square with Raspberry Coulis

FOR THE CHOCOLATE SQUARE:

1/3 cup sugar

1/3 cup maple syrup

1/4 cup vegetable oil

1/4 cup dry prunes, pureed in a blender (about 12 prunes)

1 tablespoon vanilla extract

2 eggs

2/3 cup white whole wheat flour

2/3 cup quick old-fashioned oats, ground to a flour in a blender

1/3 cup cacao powder

1/2 teaspoon baking powder

1/4 teaspoon salt

3 tablespoons water

FOR THE COULIS:

2 cups fresh raspberries

1 teaspoon lemon juice

1/4 cup maple syrup

For the chocolate square:

1. Preheat the oven to 350°F. Grease a pan (8 1/2 x 9 1/2 inch) with canola oil.
2. Beat in the sugar, maple syrup, oil, pureed prunes, and vanilla extract.
3. Add one egg at a time, constantly mixing until well incorporated.
4. Add the flour, oat flour, cacao powder, baking powder, and salt, and mix until all incorporated.
5. Mix in the water and transfer to the prepared baking dish. Bake for 20 to 25 minutes. The square is cooked when a pin inserted in the center comes out dry. Remove from oven and let cool in the pan.

For the coulis:

1. Place the raspberries in a blender, and add the lemon juice and maple syrup. Mix until smooth and thin out with a little water, if necessary. Pass through a sieve to remove seeds. Refrigerate and serve cold with the chocolate squares.

   ▸ *You may replace 2 eggs with 4 egg whites.*
   ▸ *The chocolate square may be frozen up to 1 month.*

YIELD: 16 SERVINGS

138 Cal (25% from Fat, 6% from Protein, 69% from Carb);
2 g Protein; 4 g Tot Fat; 1 g Sat Fat; 1 g Mono Fat; 25 g Carb; 2 g Fiber; 14 g Sugar; 28 mg Calcium; 1 mg Iron; 61 mg Sodium; 0 mg Cholesterol

Thin Apple Tart

3 ounces flour

2 ounces old-fashioned oats

1/2 teaspoon cinnamon

Pinch of salt

3 tablespoons canola oil

1 tablespoon vanilla

2 to 3 tablespoons water

2 large apples (about 12 ounces)

2 tablespoons apricot preserves

1. Preheat the oven to 475°F.
2. Place the oats in a blender and reduce to a flour consistency. Place the flours in a bowl.
3. Add the cinnamon, salt, oil, and vanilla, and mix until crumbly.
4. Add 1 tablespoon water at a time and continue until the dough is smooth and sticks together as one ball. Lay the dough on wax paper and push down with your palm to flatten a bit. Roll out the dough to a round thin form. Turn over the dough to a cookie sheet. Brush 1 tablespoon apricot preserves all over the pie dough surface.
5. Peel and cut the apples in half. Core, quarter, and thinly slice the apples. Starting at the edge of the dough and working inward toward the center, arrange the apple slices in overlapping circles. Finish with another circle of apple slices in the center. Bake for 15 to 20 minutes until golden brown with slightly darker edges. Heat 1 tablespoon apricot preserves with a little water to thin out in the microwave. Remove the tart from the oven and brush with the apricot preserves. Transfer the tart to a cooling rack.

YIELD: 8 SERVINGS

160 Cal (36% from Fat, 8% from Protein, 56% from Carb);
3 g Protein; 6 g Tot Fat; 1 g Sat Fat; 3 g Mono Fat; 23 g Carb; 2 g Fiber; 8 g Sugar; 38 mg Calcium; 1 mg Iron; 13 mg Sodium; 3 mg Cholesterol

Maintaining Your Park Avenue Persona

Remember our discussion of the ancient Greeks and their colorful word *diaitasthai*? Now you too understand that the word "lifestyle" means much more than that outdated definition of "diet." How about some additional wisdom from the famous Greek philosopher Aristotle? "Personal beauty is a greater recommendation than any letter of reference."

Over the past six weeks you have learned not only about beauty but also about your own self-concept. During this brief period, you have been immersed in a high-intensity program, learning how your self-concept influences your image and vice-versa. You have changed from the inside out and the outside in.

We spend many years at home, in school, and in our communities learning about the outside world, experiencing life, and forming relationships. Rarely do we focus as much attention inwardly, taking inventory, and considering how others perceive us. That's exactly what you have accomplished, so take a bow. Hopefully, you will never look at or think of yourself the same way again.

Development of one's self-concept is thought to begin around age two, when a child starts to follow a somewhat independent behavior pattern. This begins a lifelong struggle between "us" and "them," an unending challenge that may periodically seem frustrating, paralyzing, or impossible to resolve.

On the other hand, there is plenty of happiness to be discovered around us as well. Professional advancement can occur in the most unusual ways. And you need not be reminded of the uncontrollable gush of overwhelming feelings when someone appealing takes an interest in you. Thank Nature and our mysterious hormones for this phenomenon, which is capable of happening at almost any point in life.

The passage of time, advancement in the scholastic world, workplace experiences, and social interactions can affect us in both immediate and delayed ways. Our vista of life is always changing, and learning how to adapt and flourish becomes increasingly important as we ponder career opportunities and develop relationships that have the potential to last a lifetime.

That said, a necessary skill in our changing lives must be continuous insight into how we appear and how we behave. We must be capable of evolving and open to improvement, periodically reevaluating what we look like, how we present ourselves, and therefore the way the outside world sees us. Our external trappings will certainly change: hairstyles, fashion, and worldly philosophy may be rooted in a particular era. Fashion is a fickle creature, but your own style is what eventually stays.

This is neither vanity nor self-centeredness: it is a survival technique that allows us to move through various chapters of life gracefully, happily, and fearlessly. Though we prefer to avoid the thought, road blocks in our life path are an unfortunate reality, presenting us with an emotional, philosophical, and sometimes physical obstacle course. The more resilient we are, the more we know ourselves, and the more strength we possess, the better equipped we are to understand, anticipate, and transcend these problems.

People who have developed an insightful attitude toward their image have a checklist of sorts that is recounted daily. You now are capable of doing the same, having experienced an overview of the most important components of appearance and behavior, presented to you by renowned experts with years of accrued wisdom and personal success. The keys to perfecting and balancing the components of your image are now in your hands.

Most importantly, you've seen that there is no single component of image that exists in a vacuum, unaffected by the others. An interrelationship exists amongst these multiple areas that leads to a whole greater than the sum of its parts. Even a trait like self-confidence is not exclusively directed inwardly. As Dr. Krippner has taught us, "a self-confident person takes an interest in other people, in community events, in world affairs, and even in politics and spiritual issues"—in other words, it overlaps with an overall improvement in your interpersonal skills.

Conversely, interpersonal skills must reflect a person's own sense of purpose and stature. Tinsley Mortimer has described this in a most succinct and powerful way: "Good behavior must emanate from good feelings, about others and about yourself." We cannot use one set of values for ourselves and another for everyone else: this inconsistency imposes barriers to personal and professional relationships rather than fostering empathy and affection.

Perhaps you thought of makeup as a purely superficial technique of image enhancement, but that's not Laura Geller's philosophy: "It should never be obvious yet it must reflect and enhance our positive inner feelings." Moreover, she adds, "Approach makeup as an accessory to your wardrobe."

This is mirrored precisely by Joel Warren's feeling that "Your overall appearance can be broken down into several elements: hair, makeup, clothing, and jewelry. You cannot neglect one and overemphasize the others."

To this Helene Hellsten adds that the focus should never be on any component of image, as in the case of inappropriately colorful outfits: "Why attract attention to a bright outfit instead of to yourself? The trick is to look like you made no effort to dress." *You* should be the focus of attention, a confident, eloquent and poised person that commands admiration and respect from others.

Can your thinking influence your bodily physique? It must, according to Bernadette Penotti: "What you focus on grows." Concentration on form, proper breathing, and counting must be part of a successful exercise routine, especially one as time-efficient and beneficial as the one you've learned. Getting in touch with your own body is an educational experience in itself, a prelude to a lifestyle where walking tall is a constant indication to others of who you are and how you value good health.

And, to sustain your good health and exciting life, you've learned how to eat elegantly, healthfully, and carefully. Though you may have initiated this program with the sole intention of losing weight, you now have enhanced skills and insights into multiple components of your image. Why would anyone settle for just one?

And why would you want to revert to the way you were previously? Making new friends, developing deeper relationships, achieving personal success, and making a difference in your community all depend on your presentational skills, your sense of style, and, of course, on how you look. Never settle for anything less than your best, and always be ready for an upgrade. What's wrong with getting even better?

REFERENCES

Health Implications of Obesity

1. National Health and Nutrition Examination Survey (NHANES) data on the Prevalence of Overweight and Obesity among Adults-United States, 2003-2004.

2. A Potential Decline in Life Expectancy in the United States in the 21st Century, *New England Journal of Medicine,* Volume 352:1138-1145, March 17, 2005, Number 11.

3. Obesity in adulthood and its consequences for life expectancy: *Annals of Internal Medicine,* 2003, Vol. 138: 24-32.

4. Obesity and Unhealthy Life-Years in Adult Finns, *Archives of Internal Medicine 2004; 164:1413-1420.*

5. Midlife Body Mass Index and Hospitalization and Mortality in Older Age, JAMA, January 11, 2006, Vol. 295:190-198, No. 2.

6. Deaths Attributable to Obesity, *JAMA,* April 20, 2005-Vol. 293, No. 15.

7. Relation of Body Mass Index in Young Adulthood and Middle Age to Medicare Expenditures in Older Age, *JAMA,* December 2, 2004-Vol. 292, No. 22.

8. Overweight, obesity, and mortality in a large prospective cohort of persons 50 to 71 years old. Adams KF, Schatzkin, *New England Journal of Medicine* 2006;355:763-78 [PMID: 16926275]

9. Years of life lost due to obesity. Fontaine KR, Redden DT, JAMA. 2003; 289:187-93 [PMID:12517229]

10. Obesity in adulthood and its consequences for life expectancy: a life-table analysis. NEDCOM, the Netherlands Epidemiology and Demography Compression of Morbidity Research Group. *Annals of Internal Medicine.* 2003;138:24-32 [PMID: 12513041]

11. Excess deaths associated with underweight, overweight, and obesity. Flegal KM, JAMA. 2005;293:1861-7. [PMID:12513041]

12. The Obesity Epidemic in the United States—Gender, Age, Socioeconomic, Racial/Ethnic, and Geographic Characteristics: A Systematic Review and Meta-Regression Analysis. Youfa Wang and May A. Beydoun *Epidemiologic Reviews* 2007 29(1):6-28

13. Childhood Obesity What It Means for Physicians, Risa Lavizzo-Mourey, MD, MBA, *JAMA,* August 22/29, 2007-Vol 298, No.8

14. Health-related quality of life in severely obese children and adolescents. Schwimmer JB, Burwinkle TM, Varni JW. *JAMA.* 2003;289 (14):1813-1819.

15. Long-term morbidity and mortality of overweight adolescents. Must A, Jacques PF, Dallal GE, et al. *New England Journal of Medicine.* 1992;327 (19):1350-1355.

16. National medical spending attributable to overweight and obesity: how much and who's paying? Finkelstein EA, Fiebelkorn IC, Wang G. *Health Aff (Millwood).* 2003;(suppl Web exclusive):W3-219-226.

17. Overweight and obesity threaten US health gains. Satcher D; US Department of Health and Human Services. http://www.surgeongeneral.gov/topics/obesity/. Accessed June 22, 2007.

Visceral Fat, Insulin Resistance, and the Metabolic syndrome

18. The atherogenic lipoprotein profile associated with obesity and insulin resistance is largely attributable to intra-abdominal fat. Nieves D, Cnop M, Retzlaff B, et al. *Diabetes.* 2003;52:172-179.

19. Masuzaki H. et al. (2001) A transgenic model of visceral obesity and the metabolic syndrome. *Science* 294(5549), 2166-70.

20. The metabolically obese, normal-weight individual revised. *Diabetes.* 1998:47:699-713.

21. Portal adipose tissue as a generator of risk factors for cardiovascular disease and diabetes. *Arteriosclerosis.* 1990:10:493-496.

22. The Metabolic Syndrome, Inflammation and Risk of Cognitive Decline, *JAMA,* November 10, 2004-Vol. 292, No. 18.

23. Obesity, Body Fat Distribution, and Insulin Resistance, *Hypertension Primer,* American Heart Association 1999, Pages 256-258.

24. Adipose tissue as an endocrine organ, Kershaw EE, Flier JS. *J Clin Endocrinol Metab. 2004;89: 2548-2556.*

25. Obesity and the role of adipose tissue in inflammation and metabolism, Greenberg AS, Obin MS. *American Journal of Clinical Nutrition.* 2006;83: 461S-465S.

Obesity as a Risk Factor for Illness

26. Is Obesity a Factor for More Aggressive Prostate Cancer, Disease Recurrence? *Journal of Clinical Oncology,* February 2004, Medical College of Georgia and Veterans Affairs Medical Center in Augusta.

27. The obesity-hypoventilation syndrome, *American Journal of Medicine,* 2005, Vol. 118, Pages 948-956.

28. Researchers Consider Possible Mechanistic Links between Obesity and Asthma; *Journal of Allergy and Clinical Immunology* May 2005.

29. Obesity and the risk of breast cancer *Wall Street Journal* 2/26/04, data from American Cancer Society.

30. Obesity and the Risk of New-Onset Atrial Fibrillation, *JAMA*, November 24, 2004-Vol. 292, No. 20.

31. Insulin Resistance and Risk of Congestive Heart Failure, *JAMA*, July 20, 2005-Vol. 294, 3.

32. Obesity, Weight Gain, and the Risk of Kidney Stones, *JAMA*, January 26, 2005-Vol. 293, 4.

33. Effect of a multidisciplinary program of weight reduction on endothelial functions in obese women, *Journal of Endocrinological Investigation,* 2003, vol. 26, n°3, pp. RC5-RC8.

34. Type II diabetes in children and adolescents. American Diabetes Association. *Pediatrics.* 2000; 105(3pt 1):671-680.

The Dietary Approach to Obesity

35. The Dietary Approach to Obesity. Is It the Diet or the Disorder? Editorial in *JAMA*, January 5, 2005; Vol. 293, No.1.

36. What works for obesity? *British Medical Journal* monograph, April 30, 2004.

37. The truth about low-carb foods, *Consumer Reports*, June 2004.

38. A Low-Carbohydrate, Ketogenic Diet versus a Low-Fat Diet to Treat Obesity and Hyperlipidemia; *Annals of Internal Medicine:* May 18, 2004, Volume 140, Issue 10:769-777.

39. Comparison of the Atkins, Ornish, Weight Watchers, and Zone Diets for Weight Loss and Heart Disease Risk Reduction. *JAMA*, January 5, 2005 – Vol. 293, No.1.

40. Popular diets: correlation to health, nutrition, and obesity. *Journal of the American Dietetic Association.* 2001 Apr;101(4):411-20.

41. Commercial Weight-Loss Programs: Little Evidence, *Journal Watch Cardiology*, February 11, 2005; 2005(211).

42. Systematic Review: An Evaluation of Major Commercial Weight Loss Programs in the United States, *Annals of Internal Medicine*, January 4, 2005, Vol. 142, Issue 1:56-66.

43. Atkins and other low-carbohydrate diets: hoax or an effective tool for weight loss? *The Lancet* 2004, Vol. 364: 897-99.

44. Comparison of the Atkins, Zone, Ornish, and LEARN Diets for Change in Weight and Related Risk Factors among Overweight Premenopausal Women: The A TO Z Weight Loss Study: A Randomized Trial Christopher D. Gardner; Alexandre Kiazand; Sofiya Alhassan; Soowon Kim; Randall S. Stafford; Raymond R. Balise; Helena C. Kraemer; Abby C. King *JAMA*, March 7, 2007; 297: 969-977.

45. Meta-analysis: The Effect of Dietary Counseling for Weight Loss; Michael L. Dansinger, MD, MS, *Annals of Internal Medicine*, July 3, 2007, Volume 147 Number 1, Page 41-50.

Related Topics

46. Fast food intake among adolescents; *JAMA*, June 16, 2004-Vol. 291, No. 23.

47. Sugar-Sweetened Soft Drinks, Obesity, and Type 2 Diabetes; *JAMA*, August 25, 2004-Vol 292, No. 8.

48. Green Tea and Obese Zucker Rats: Incer, Kaliebe, Porter and Svec, Unpublished, 2003.

49. Soft Drink Consumption and Risk of Developing Cardiometabolic Risk Factors and the Metabolic Syndrome in Middle-Aged Adults in the Community, Ravi Dhingra et al, *Circulation*, July 23, 2007: 107:481-488

50. Harrison's *Principles of Internal Medicine*, 16th edition, McGraw Hill 2005.

References Part 2.

1. Csikszentmihalyi, M. (1993). *The Evolving Self: A Psychology for the Third Millennium*. New York: Harper Collins.

2. Ellis, A. (2004). *The Road to Tolerance: The Philosophy of Rational Emotive Behavior Therapy*. Amherst, NY: Prometheus Books.

3. Feinstein, D. and Krippner. S. (2006). The Mythic Path (3rd edition of *Personal Mythology: The Psychology of Your Evolving Self*). Santa Rosa, CA: Elite Books.

4. LeShan, L. (1974). *How to Meditate: A Guide to Self-discovery*. Boston: Little, Brown.

5. Mann, T. et al. (2007). Medicare's search for effective obesity treatments: *Diets are not the answer*. American Psychologist, Volume 62, pages 220-233.

6. Park, D (Editor). (April, 2007). *Eating Disorders*. A Special Issue of the American Psychologist. Washington, DC: American Psychological Association.

7. Seligman, M. (1998). *Learned Optimism*. New York: Free Press.

8. Ellis, A. (2005). *The Myth of Self-Esteem*. Amherst, N.Y. Prometheus Books

9. Krippner, S., & Ryan, C. (2001). Food in the Neolithic Age. In R.-I. Heinze (Ed.), *Proceedings of the Nineteenth Annual Conference on the Study of Shamanism and Alternate Modes of Healing* (pp. 217-219). Berkeley, CA: Independent Scholars of Asia.

10. Rudolf, H. and Morrison, C. (2008). *The Brain, Appetite, and Obesity*. Annual Review of Psychology, Vol. 59, pages 55–91.

INDEX